MOM, MANIA, and ME

Surviving and Changing a Volatile Relationship

Mom, Mania, and Me: Surviving and Changing a Volatile Relationship
Copyright 2017 ©Diane Dweller
All rights reserved
Published in the United States
Writing Ink L.L.C.
Tucson, Arizona

This publication contains the personal account of the author who is not rendering psychological or professional services in this book. It is intended to provide helpful and informative material on the subject matter covered. If the reader requires expert or medical assistance, personal counseling or advice, a competent professional should be consulted. The author specifically disclaims any responsibility for any liability, loss or risk, personal or otherwise, which is incurred as a consequence, directly or indirectly in the use or application of any of the contents of this book.

ISBN 978-0-944749-02-9
ebook ISBN 978-0-944749-00-5
Library of Congress Control Number: 2016905656

    Dweller, Diane, author.
      Mom, mania, and me : surviving and changing a
    volatile relationship / Diane Dweller.
      pages cm
      Includes bibliographical references.
      LCCN 2016905656
      ISBN 978-0-944749-02-9 (paperback)
      ISBN 978-0-944749-00-5 (ebook)
      1. Dweller, Diane. 2. Children of mentally ill
    mothers--United States--Biography. 3. Manic-depressive
    illness--Popular works. 4. Adult child abuse victims--
    United States--Biography. 5. Autobiographies.
    I. Title.
    RC516.D94 2016   616.89'5
              QBI16-900018

To the best of her ability, the author has re-created events, locales and conversations from her memories of them in a way that evokes the feeling and meaning of the true events. In order to maintain the anonymity of others, the names of places and individuals, including the author, have been changed.

To order bulk copies, discounted class sets, or to arrange a media interview, please visit DianeDweller.com

Book design by StoriesToTellBooks.com

MOM, MANIA, and ME

Surviving and Changing
a Volatile Relationship

DIANE DWELLER

Contents

Prologue		1
1	Three Decades Later	3
2	Unexpected Help	15
3	Earliest Memories	26
4	Frantic Survival	37
5	Mom's Spells	51
6	Mom's Help	62
7	Teen Angst: Confrontation # 1	68
8	Escaping from Mom	84
9	Cold Anger: Confrontation # 2	95
10	Starting Over	107
11	Epiphanies: Changing Myself	119
12	Good Things Happen	130
13	Chemical Turmoil	141
14	Diagnosis and Hallelujahs	147
15	Compliance Challenges	154
16	Sad Anger: Confrontation # 3	163
17	Doing Something Right	172
18	Questions: Confrontation # 4	182
19	Gracie: Confrontation # 5	190
20	Tragedy, Love, Peace	197
Epilogue		209
Appendix		211
	Facts and Data about Mental Illness	213
	Bipolar Disorder Information and Resources	218
A Conversation with Author Diane Dweller		221
Book Club Discussion Questions		225
Acknowledgments		227

Prologue

"NOW STAY THERE AND DON'T move," I whisper to Bitsy as she curls up next to me under the dining room table. Her brown and white tail is tickling my leg. I try not to giggle.

I like to play under the table. The long white tablecloth makes a safe cave. And there are two doorways. I can escape to the kitchen or the living room.

I pick up my doll Mary and start to pull on the pink dress she wants to wear today.

Bitsy's ears perk up. Footsteps. In the kitchen. I put my hand on her head, gently holding her down.

Louder steps. She's coming this way. Can I escape?

I see Mom's white high heels coming through the doorway.

Too late. I freeze. I can't breathe. I gasp for air.

Did she hear me?

Don't find me. Don't find me.

She's coming toward my hiding place. My tummy hurts. I try to breathe quieter through my mouth. Too loud.

The shoes stop next to the table.

I stop breathing.

1

Three Decades
Later

"Diane's here."

"She's here."

The quiet whisper swept through the mass of mourners gathered in my parents' living room as I entered the front door. A path silently opened as I passed through the crowd searching among them for Mom, my stomach churning.

My steps slowed when I saw her framed in the doorway at the end of the hall, her slim figure silhouetted against the lights of the back bedroom. She stood still, expressionless, but then reached out with both arms as I drew near.

Our arms tentatively encircled each other. As her head came to rest on my shoulder, her arms tightened around my ribs—tighter and tighter—reducing my breaths to shallow pants. I could feel the rhythmic thump of my pounding heart against her cheek. The lump in my throat blocked all words. Our breaths intermingled as we clung to each other in this unexpected embrace, silently sharing our grief.

The next morning Mom breezed into her sunny yellow kitchen, neatly groomed in a navy pant suit with a matching purse over her arm. "We need to go to the funeral home and make sure everything is done properly." She silently eyed each of the four of us sitting around the breakfast room table.

I glanced at Alex and Andrea, my two teenagers who had come with me from Vancouver. Both stared at me with alarm. Barely awake and still in pajamas, they obviously hoped I would not insist they go.

"We need to go." Mom looked at my sister Gracie. "Now."

Gracie, my only sibling, shook her head. "I'd rather not go. I want to remember Dad as he was alive." Gracie's family of five had driven the three hours to North Creek soon after Mom's midnight call to each of us with the shocking news of Dad's death. During my twelve-hour, multi-layover trip from Canada to Texas, my organized older sister had helped Mom choose the casket, select Dad's burial clothes, plan the service, and greet the gathering family.

Turning my way, Mom asked, "What about you?"

"I'll go," I said. Maybe it would help me accept this tragedy. I slipped out of my chair and headed toward the garage. "I'll drive," I called out over my shoulder, trying to get to the car before she did.

"Okay, but put on some lipstick."

Easing into the driver's seat, I discovered Mom still left her car keys in the ignition in the open, unlocked garage. As she climbed into the passenger's seat the syrupy scent of White Shoulders perfume filled the car. I cracked my window.

Maneuvering the heavy Buick down broad familiar streets, I observed what had once been a thriving Texas town. Shrugging, trying to shake off exhaustion, I turned left past the Dairy Queen and noticed how drought had ravaged the small town. Glaring sun beat down on tired houses; paint peeled off porches like a bad sunburn. Empty windows and bare yards spoke of years of hard times. Yet, here and there, patches of green grass added a touch of spring to the dun-colored terrain.

Mom uttered not a word for several minutes—no gossipy chatter about people I didn't know or want to hear about.

Her silence didn't last.

"I hope you like the casket color. We picked out a blue one. His favorite color. It costs too much. Too darn much. They get you in there and overwhelm you and you have to decide right then, and it's too much. They make you feel guilty if you ask about a cheaper one. And a casket isn't enough. You feel like you have to buy a vault too, and on and on. It shouldn't cost so much. I told them we are not going to have an open casket funeral. Having people file by to look at Edward's body is barbaric. Just barbaric. Besides, it would take too long.

"Oh look at Martha's forsythia. I've never seen them so loaded with blooms. Mine almost didn't make it through all the freezes this winter.

Should have mulched them better. Did you notice Rebecca's hair last night? It looked awful. What did you bring to wear to the funeral?

I hope you didn't bring black. I can't decide what to wear. Definitely not black. Not black."

Not a tear. Not a word about Dad or his death. Obviously in denial, Mom acted like nothing tragic had occurred. Her fast talking was starting to scare me. Please, please don't have a spell. I can't cope with your problem right now.

Heat shimmered above the hot pavement as I turned the car into the parking lot in front of the white, sprawling, two-story house that served as a funeral home. Mom hopped out and at a brisk pace headed for the cool interior. I hustled and followed her inside, blinking as my eyes adjusted to the subdued interior lighting. I recognized the faint strain of a familiar hymn, the words promising a life beyond the grave.

"Dixie. Diane." The tall funeral director, one of my dad's best friends, gestured to a side room. "Edward's in here, Dixie. I'll close the doors to give you privacy as long as you need it. I'll be right here if you want anything."

As Mom entered the room, he put his arm around my shoulders and whispered, "Diane, thank goodness you're here. Dixie's going to need you more than ever."

I nodded, feeling shaky, unable to cope with this moment—much less Mom's problem.

I looked up as we entered the viewing room, taking in the steel-blue casket and Dad's body, but not his death. I felt light-headed. This is surreal. He's too young. We need him here. Mom needs him. This wasn't supposed to happen. Not yet. I felt much too young at thirty-six to be burying my dad.

Mom reached out and patted the arm of his blue suit as she looked at the body of the love-of-her-life, her husband of forty years. "Everything looks fine. Even his hands."

I looked at Dad's long tapered fingers, his always immaculate nails. So still now. Hands that had tossed me in the air. Hands that had delicately moved a surgeon's scalpel to separate diseased tissue from healthy. Hands that had held many of the citizens in this town as they gasped their first breath of life.

Mom's composure confused me.

She had not exhibited any sign of being upset, tearful or mournful. I realized that she must be in either a state of shock or denial, or both.

Mom's attention strayed to the numerous floral tributes for a few moments, then with a last glance at Dad and a curt nod, she said, "Everything's fine. Let's go." She headed for the door.

"Go?" I couldn't breathe. I needed to sit down. I lingered, looking at the anchor of my life, the rock who held our family together. I felt my heart steady, a calmness settle over me as I realized that, yes, it is his body but he isn't in it anymore. His spirit is free.

I wanted to spend some quiet time saying my final goodbye, to begin accepting his death, but Mom had already disappeared and I knew better than to let her get in the driver's seat.

I'll grieve later, I thought. When I get back to Canada. With a quick last glance at Dad, I turned and left.

As I exited the funeral home, I caught sight of Mom talking to a tall, heavy-set man out on the sidewalk. She looked much younger than sixty-six, and still very attractive. Her natural dark brown hair held nary a sign of any gray. Approaching them, I heard her don't-mess-with-me voice, "Twenty minutes. Not a minute longer or I'll get up and walk out." The man nodded assurance, said something, then passed me heading for the funeral home entrance.

"Hurry. Get in and turn on the air conditioner," Mom demanded. "Cool off this car."

"Who was that?" I asked, digging in my purse for the keys.

"Our new preacher. I told him not to talk more than twenty minutes. That church is going to be full and you get a Baptist preacher with the biggest congregation he's ever had and he won't know when to hush."

I blinked and wondered: Does this new preacher know Mom really will get up and walk out of her own husband's funeral if he talks too long?

Opening the car door, I heard a shout, "Yoo-hoo! Dixie, Diane." Jessie, the undertaker's wife and Mom's good friend waved as she walked toward us across the lawn next door, apron flapping in the Texas wind. "Diane, we're so glad you got here safely. This has been so sudden, such a shock to us all," she said, enveloping me in a bear hug. "Are Rex and the children with you? We'd love to have your family stay here with us."

"Alex and Andrea did come, but Rex needed to stay in Vancouver to take care of Shannon who is still recovering from scarlet fever. She is just three and we didn't think it safe for her to travel yet."

Turning, Jessie said, "Dixie, then we want some of your other family members to come and stay with us. And I have a large ham in the oven and some cornbread I'll be bringing over shortly."

Hmmmm. Cornbread. I was definitely back in the South.

WE RETURNED TO A HOUSE full of family and friends and a growing number of floral arrangements that filled the air with sweet fragrance. Later, just as Gracie started to organize items for lunch, the back doorbell rang again. In trooped five church women loaded with platters of fried chicken, green beans, sweet potato casserole with marshmallows on the top, gelatin salads, biscuits and gravy. Where were they going to find space in the kitchen? Bedlam threatened, but within seconds, they had the kitchen well under control. When lunch was ready, more than twenty people, mostly out-of-town relatives, lined up for an extensive buffet in the dining area of the den.

MOM SAT STARING AT HER barely touched food, then said, "Diane, I want to go do something. Will you help me?" She rose from the table.

"Sure. What are we going to do?" I followed her into the crowded kitchen.

"Dixie, is everything all right?" a helper asked.

"Yes, it's wonderful. Thank you. Thank you all for coming. The food is delicious. We have so much. Here Diane, help me wrap up the rest of Jessie's ham. I want to take it to the Wordalls."

"To Dr. Wordall's? Why?"

"We've had a big loss, but so have they. Their daughter had a wreck last night and their precious three-year-old granddaughter was thrown from the car and killed. And I want to go see them."

Daddy just died and she is thinking of how she can help someone else in their grief. How like her, always wanting to help others, to share what she has, even at this moment. Busy hands stilled. Silence settled over the kitchen as Mom wrapped the ham in tinfoil. First one of the helpers and then another reached for a tissue.

Life isn't fair. Neither is death.

It was not the custom in the South in the 1970s to have a formal visitation time for a family to receive friends at the funeral home. As a result, after we returned from the Wordall's an unending troupe of people continued to arrive at our house all day and all evening. Each chime of the doorbell brought another memory into the house: my third grade teacher, Dad's golfing buddy, Garden Club ladies, doctors from the clinic and florists bearing more and more flowers. People and floral arrangements crowded the large den that we already called the jungle room due to Mom's fifteen house plants scattered among the rattan chairs, love seats and tables. Additional arrangements now lined the chartreuse-colored walls and were clumped together in a corner on the brown Mexican tile floor.

A long-time friend of the family touched me on the arm. Gesturing to her husband, she asked, "Diane, could we talk to you privately for a moment?"

"Yes, of course." We retreated to a quiet area next to the fireplace in the formal living room. I turned to face them, curious to know what they wanted to say in private.

"Diane, we want to know what we can do to help when Dixie has one of her spells," she said.

Stunned, I glanced from her to her husband.

Her husband added, "Edward talked to me many times about Dixie's spells and that it was getting harder and harder to help her through them. What can we do to help now that he's gone?"

I felt tears stinging my eyes. This was the first time anyone outside the family had acknowledged to me that they knew about Mom's "little problem" as she described it. And they wanted to help.

If only they could.

"Oh how I wish I knew the answer," I said, shaking my head. "Gracie and I don't know what to do. The fear of what Mom may do now that Dad isn't here to settle her down is keeping me awake nights. I live so far away and it takes Gracie several hours to get here."

I stared into space, glimpsing the chaos that lay ahead. After thinking a moment, I said, "I guess the best thing you could do is to call one of us when you see any signs that she is starting to get hyper. Please call one of us if she starts calling you over and over, or talking incessantly or driving too fast. The sooner we know, the better. We might be able to stop her before it's too late."

Three Decades Later 9

I knew that if we weren't notified soon enough, Mom would lose control of her impulses, have another wreck—possibly injuring herself or killing someone—or take off on another extravagant spending spree.

And when they call, what are we supposed to do? How can we stop the unstoppable Dixie? A feeling of hopelessness enveloped me.

BY TEN O'CLOCK THAT EVENING, my eyelids were drooping as low as my spirits. Conversation among the group of relatives still seated in the den wafted over me, blurring into distant hums. My head tilted. I jerked awake, looking to see if anyone noticed.

Mom looked exhausted too. Gracie and her family had already gone to the motel. Finally, breaching southern hospitality, I stood up and reached out to help Mom up. Turning to the others, I said, "Please excuse us."

Mom looked confused. "Where are we going?"

"To bed. You need to rest for the funeral tomorrow." As we stood up, so did the guests, taking my hint, saying they needed to leave. After the front door closed, Mom headed to her bedroom and I to the kitchen to tidy it up.

"Please take one of those sleeping pills the doctor gave you," I called out to her. "We all need to sleep good tonight."

Twenty minutes later I peeked into Mom's bedroom to check on her. She lifted her head up off the pillow, beckoned to me and patted the bed next to her. I stretched out beside her, not sure what she wanted.

She mumbled something as she turned on her side toward me. I didn't answer. Her eyes closed. Minutes ticked by.

"Mumble, mumble. Jack ... came ... interested in me."

What's she talking about? I wondered.

She paused, then continued, " I look ... like wife ... died."

What is she thinking? Dad's not even buried and she thinks some widower is hot for her?

"Jack ... nice looking," she murmured.

Good grief. I can't stay here listening to this.

I slipped out of her bed and headed for the guest room. Too weary to even brush my teeth, I undressed and crawled into bed, only to toss for hours wondering what Gracie and I could do to stop Mom's next spell.

I AWAKENED TO SUNSHINE STREAMING through the sheer curtains. I held one aside and peered out. It was not a funeral-type of day. Puffy clouds dotted the cerulean sky. Birds of all types were calling for mates, mockingbirds trilling their musical score of stolen melodies. Leaves were budding on the bare mesquite tree limbs and yellow daffodils swayed in the wind, signaling a time for life to awaken, not end.

By mid-morning we were all dressed in our funeral clothes. I had on my navy suit and high heels making me several inches taller than Gracie. We did look like sisters, sharing deep-set hazel eyes and high cheekbones, but our coloring differed. Gracie had thick, wavy dark-auburn hair. A few pale freckles dotted her fair cheeks. I had sun-streaked light brown hair and a tan that deepened daily.

I heard the jingle of the charm bracelet Dad had given Mom before I entered the breakfast room where our immediate family had gathered. Mom had decided on a light blue dress. She looked fretful, agitated.

The black limos arrived to collect the family. The main driver announced it was time to go.

"Gracie," Mom turned, her arms fluttering in the air, alarm in her voice, "Where is that big photograph of Edward that hung in the hospital lobby that you brought home? I wanted that placed in front of the casket."

The driver from the funeral home looking at his watch. He raised his eyebrows at me.

"Mom, we need to leave," I said. "The service will be fine without the picture."

"No, we are going to take it. Find it. NOW."

Several of us scattered, frantically looking. "Here it is," Gracie called from the laundry room.

"Take it to the church," Mom demanded, looking at the driver. "I want it right next to the casket so everybody can see him."

"Mrs. Dweller, we can take it with us when you go," the driver suggested.

"No. Take it now," she said in her don't-mess-with-me-voice. "Come back for us. They won't start without us there."

He left with the picture.

Twenty minutes later the extended family crowded into three limousines for the short ride to the First Baptist Church. Police were still waving cars into the crowded parking lots. The American, Texas and Christian flags flew at half-mast in Dad's honor.

As we waited in the foyer, a kaleidoscope of memories clicked through my mind. For forty years my dad had been a beloved physician and civic leader in this small town. Patients loved Dad's pragmatic style of country doctoring. He believed in treating the whole patient including emotional issues, often finding clues to physical illnesses in this area. Sympathy cards and letters were filled with wonderful personal stories of how he had birthed them, healed them, operated on them—when no one else would take the chance—saved their lives, and sometimes their marriages.

Organ music swelled and ebbed as we entered the sanctuary. Not funeral dirges. Mom had insisted on robust hymns like "Shall We Gather at the River" and "When We All Get to Heaven." With Mom leading, head held high, the extended family walked down the long aisle toward the reserved front pews. In the two-story church nave, banks of floral arrangements surrounded the closed casket. People filled every pew on the huge main floor. Glancing up at the balcony, I saw people still in the aisles, looking for a seat. Hundreds had come to pay their respects.

Walking behind Mom, trying to deny the reality of the moment, I felt tears I'd choked down for days, threatening to spill over. Keep yourself together a little longer Diane, I chided myself, biting my cheek. Mom will be upset if you break down or embarrass her.

I felt a wail building inside of me. What is so shameful about showing that my heart is broken? I wanted to throw myself on the casket keening to release my anguish, to wail like mourners in other cultures. I struggled to keep from breaking into uncontrollable sobs as Mom's mantra echoed in my head. What will people say?

Manners prevailed. I sat down, outwardly composed. Inside I raged, angry not only at death, but also at the stiff-upper-lip behavior our society and my mother expected. I longed for my husband's presence and comfort. I needed him, but knew our sick three year old did too.

I tried focusing on Dad's large photograph taken a year earlier, now displayed next to the casket. It showed how young he still looked at age sixty-six. How vital. It belied the damage to his heart that caused this unexpected funeral.

The music crested. A hush descended over the sanctuary. The pastor began the eulogy revealing many anecdotes of how frequently my father had helped others, often without anyone else being aware of it, including Mom.

He kept it short. Nineteen minutes short. Somebody must have clued him in.

A final prayer and we were ushered out, back into the limos to be driven to the cemetery at the slowest pace that wide-open Texas highway had ever seen. By the time we arrived and gathered under the tent, the casket and flowers had been placed beside the open grave.

Mom motioned to the preacher. "Start the service."

"Dixie, shouldn't we wait for the other people to arrive?" he asked. I glanced back across the valley and saw miles of cars heading our way, as far as the eye could see.

"No. That will take too long. Start now."

Stunned, I wondered how she could ignore all those people or social protocol. Why was she in such a hurry? What was her rush? These people loved dad and wanted to show their respects. What will people say about this?

A lifetime of knowing how futile it was to countermand Mom's orders cemented my silence—and Gracie's.

The pastor, with a perplexed expression, stared at Mom.

"Start." She glared at him.

He started. He kept it short there too. As soon as the last "Amen" faded in the air, she announced, "Let's go." I hurried to catch up with her as she headed toward the limousine. Cars were still pouring into the cemetery. As our limousine started to move forward, I heard a rapping on the car window. It was Rob, a medical intern in Dallas and the son of close family friends. My dad had a great deal to do with his decision to become a doctor.

"Stop," I called out to the driver as I rolled the window down.

"Don't stop," Mom countered.

"Dixie, Diane, Gracie," Tom gasped, obviously out of breath as he jogged to keep up with the car, "I want to tell you how sorry I am. I've driven five hours to be here and I have to go right back." We left him standing there, exhaustion and sadness etched on his face.

I lost count of the cars headed into the cemetery as we left.

Three Decades Later 13

THE NEXT DAY GRACIE AND I slipped back into the guestroom to try to make some logical plans. I stretched out on the aqua bedspread, and rubbed my forehead, trying to smooth the lines of exhaustion. Gracie stretched out beside me with a deep sigh.

"What," I asked, "are we going to do about Mom? I can't hop back down here with twelve-hour flights each time she launches into one of her frantic alienate-everyone capers."

"I don't know," Gracie said, "Daddy never discussed what he did to get her to settle down—if she ever did. I think he just had to wait it out until her spell tapered off several weeks later. Let's hope she doesn't start a spell for a long time."

When Mom's next spell would start was always an unknown, but that another one would happen was a given.

We decided I would stay for a month to help Mom while Gracie returned home, both of us knowing she would be the one stuck with most of Mom's care in the future. I accepted my role with mixed emotions. The urge to flee from Mom, ingrained since early childhood, all but overwhelmed me.

I HAD BEEN ABLE TO keep my grief at bay when surrounded by people and actions that needed to be done, but grief is a sneak. It hits hard. Without warning. When one least expects it. Like when I went alone to the grocery store. Pushing a cart down an aisle, I felt it strike with a sucking in of air and a feeling of panic, like the air couldn't get in. Despair spilled over me, sweeping down my torso, making my legs quiver with weakness. I leaned on the cart. Unbidden tears began to flow down my cheeks. I struggled to gain the upper hand and push the pain back into my "I'll grieve-later box." I failed. Gasping for air, I noticed a little girl staring at me, her eyes wide. I forced the box open, took a deep breath, wiped my wet cheeks with the back of my hand and gave her a shaky smile.

I sniffed hard.

Tissues. Which aisle has tissues?

AFTER GRACIE LEFT, I THOUGHT Mom and I would begin to adjust to our new roles, me as helper, she as grieving widow. I started on a long list of things to do, but she slipped further into denial, acting like nothing had changed.

Actually perky, she started chattering rapidly and constantly about people, events, new restaurants, about anything but the sad gap in our lives. Then I realized she was sleeping only about four hours at night. I knew what that meant—a dreaded spell had started.

I called Gracie from Dad's office, hopeful that she could think of something.

"She is definitely starting a spell. What do you think I should do?" I asked.

"Try to get her to slow down." Gracie responded.

"How?"

"Is she still taking a nap?"

"Yeah, for all of five minutes," I said, exasperated.

"Tell her you'll wake her in half-an-hour, and to stay in bed that long and rest."

That didn't work.

When it came to Mom's spells, even Dad hadn't been able to stop her when her thoughts and actions swirled into frenzied mode. How were Gracie and I supposed to?

2

Unexpected Help

DAD'S LAWYER CAME FROM AUSTIN to read his will at our local bank. Six of us gathered around the huge walnut table in the private conference room. Mom, Gracie and her husband, and I sat on one side. The lawyer and Charles, our banker and a close family friend, sat on the other. When the attorney opened Dad's bank box, Mom spied a cache of money among the papers. Her eyes grew large as she stood up, reached into the box and started gathering up the hundred dollar bills. They became even larger when she started to put a fist full of the cash in her purse and the attorney firmly said, "Mrs. Dweller, you can't have that yet."

"What do you mean? Edward left it to me. It's mine isn't it?"

"Yes, but until the probate is complete and all debts are settled, you can't have it."

"I never heard of such, telling me I can't have what's mine. This doesn't make any sense. How am I going to pay the bills?" Deep frown lines appeared between her hazel eyes.

Charles spoke up, "Dixie, you will have plenty of money from Edward's insurance, pension and other sources and I'm here for you. You tell me what you want and I'll see to it."

"I want this money right here in my hand," she said, waving the bills at him.

"You got me there. I can't give you that money, but I can transfer the same amount to your checking account. Will that do?"

An obstinate look settled on Mom's face and I thought we were in for a stormy session, but her public manners won. With a nod and a frown, she gave up and sat down.

We all knew what Dad's will contained, so there weren't any surprises. He had placed all his assets in two living trusts to support Mom. One was

16   MOM, MANIA, AND ME

her own trust; the other was to come to Gracie and me if she remarried or after she died—if any money remained. Both trusts were to be managed by the Trust Department at a huge bank in Dallas. This trust system required Mom to formally request—and wait—for any substantial amounts she wanted for expensive purchases. Gracie and I hoped it would work to curtail her impulsive spending during her spells.

We had seen Mom blow through her generous monthly allowance in her checking account during one visit to a shopping or garden center. Since she absolutely refused to keep her checkbook balanced, Charles would call Dad several times a year and say, "Edward, she's done it again." Dad would tell him to fill her account back up. She spent. He filled. Now Mom was in charge of both spending and filling. While not wealthy, with care, Mom could live a long life very comfortably.

A sense of foreboding swept through me.

THE NEXT MORNING, THE SUN poured in through the bay windows in the breakfast room creating rectangles of light over stacks of papers scattered on the maple table. I poured myself a hot cup of coffee and sat down. Sitting across the table in her aqua robe, her hair brushed, her lipstick on, Mom picked up one page, looked at it, then me. A hint of panic darted over her face.

"I don't know how to pay this bill. I've never paid a utility bill in my life," she wailed. She started stacking and re-stacking the piles of bills and sympathy cards.

I took a sip of coffee before replying. "Sure you can."

"No, I can't. I don't know how to pay utility bills."

After a few moments of mental groaning, I thought of a comparison she might accept.

"How do you pay for the clothes you buy at Inez's or Kantor's?" I asked.

She blinked then said, "I put them on my charge cards."

"When you get the bill in the mail for the clothes you bought, what do you do?"

"I write them a check. But," she insisted, "utilities are different."

"Maybe not so different. Every time you turn on an electric light, the electric company puts it on your electricity charge card. And every month they send you a bill just like the stores do. All you have to do is write them a check, like your checks to the stores."

"But utilities aren't the same. I can't pay them," she whimpered.

How, I wondered, staring at her, can a human dynamo who takes over and runs every organization she belongs to, not feel capable of paying the electric bill? What is with this helpless woman routine?

One advantage of living in a small town is that you know who the good guys are. I called Charles at the bank and he took care of it. Long before banks and utility companies caught on to this idea, Mom's small bank started making automatic payments to her utility companies.

One hurdle cleared. At least her electricity, gas and water would not be shut off.

LATER THAT WEEK MOM CALLED the Trust Department at the bank in Dallas with some questions about the trusts Dad had set up. She left a message with the receptionist. She called again. And again. Four times that day, and the next. No response. "Why can't they call me back when I want to talk to them? I don't like it one bit. Charles always calls me immediately." A day later someone finally called back. Too late. Irritated, her ire precipitated a trip to Dallas for a face-to-face meeting with the bank officers who would be her contacts, and to hopefully establish rapport with them.

Gracie and her husband, a successful businessman, joined us on our trip to Dallas to the bank's Trust Department. Entering the skyscraper, the four of us made our serpentine way around the colossal marble pillars that bespoke affluence and tradition. The elevator ascended rapidly; ears popped to subtle classical music. We stepped out, sinking into deep carpet. In awe and silence Mom scrutinized the Midas decor of enormous oil paintings, dark walnut credenzas and gigantic floral masterpieces. She reached out, touched several flowers, then sniffed one before whispering in awe, "They're real."

Two trust officers greeted us, one tall, one short, both wearing well-tailored navy suits, white shirts and power ties. They escorted us into an office overlooking the vast Dallas skyline below. Condolences were tendered before we sat down in the plush chairs. Normally chatty, Mom took her seat, subdued and silent. Our inquiries about how she should contact them and how the trusts would be invested were met with assurances. "Our excellent investment team will see that your trusts are well invested and the principal protected."

I asked what I considered a perfectly reasonable question, "What rate of return may we expect on the investments?" A look passed between them before they repeated their general assurances. I repeated my question. Another look passed between them. Addressing only my brother-in-law the tall officer said, "The market varies and we cannot say exactly what the rate of return will be in the future."

My gut and my recently liberated hackles started zinging. Why were they so evasive?

Mom, who had remained silent through this exchange, piped up in a loud excited voice, "Tell me, do I have enough money to buy an airplane and hire a pilot?"

Five heads whipped around and stared at her in surprise.

"Buy an airplane?" Gracie and I blurted out in unison.

"Why do you want an airplane?" one trust officer asked.

"I love to travel and this would make it so much easier, so much more fun. I could call my pilot up and fly anywhere I want to, anytime."

Lordy, lordy, lordy. I could just see her. Auntie Mame herself, jetting around the world, shopping in London, Paris, Shanghai. A plane? Good grief, what else does she want to buy? How are we going to keep her from blowing through the trusts?

The taller advisor replied in a condescending tone, "Mrs. Dweller, airplanes are very expensive, not only to purchase, but also to maintain. That would not be the best investment for your size of trusts."

Mom, looking crestfallen, opened her mouth, then shut it.

Gracie tried to assure her, "You'll be able to travel in style, Mom. First class."

I turned back to the former topic they obviously wanted to avoid. "I realize you cannot predict future returns, but would you please tell us what rates of return other trusts of this size, now invested with you, have made this quarter?"

They looked at each other until the tall one gave the short one a nod. He responded quietly, "About five percent."

Unexpected Help 19

"Five percent. And what is the rate of inflation now here in the U. S.?" That resulted in a very long pause. They looked at each other, at their shoes, anywhere but at me.

"Please, tell me what it is. I live in Canada and I'm not up-to-date on the current rate of inflation here." More silence.

The tall officer finally looked at me a long moment before he replied, "About nine percent."

I blinked in astonishment. Her money would earn only five percent with inflation at nine percent. I paused before replying, "Thank you."

Between Mom's spending habits and this discrepancy she could get in serious financial trouble.

After our return to North Creek, Mom called the officers with more questions. Again it took days for them to call back. This shredded any rapport established during our trip. Mom became ticked off at them. And when ticked off, her anger often resulted in instant, regrettable actions. Concerned about what she might do after I left, Gracie and I immediately took the steps needed to switch the money to the Trust Department in a smaller bank where Gracie's husband served on the board. Mom's trusts were assigned to a wonderful woman who excelled in communicating with a widow who wanted to jet off in her own expensive private plane. Their low rate of return equaled that of most bank trust departments, but at least her calls were answered promptly. Mom loved being treated like the special client she considered herself.

Gracie said, "I'm so relieved Dad arranged the finances this way. Mom never stopped to ask him before making extravagant purchases. She just spent. This trust requires her to request and wait before getting large sums of money. Hopefully it will halt her over-spending habits."

I BECAME MORE CONCERNED AS Mom's comments and actions accelerated. Suspecting she would have trouble concentrating and completing the numerous legal tasks required by Dad's death, I took over this job. Settling his estate included finding numerous elusive documents and going over to Dad's clinic to make multiple copies in the business office.

I crossed off first one task and then another. A sense of satisfaction swept over me, but the to-do-list grew longer, not shorter, as the days went by. The date I would be leaving drew close and the challenge of Mom's irrational fear of being alone after dark had me perplexed. How do you solve a phobia?

I did the best I could to secure her home—a direct alarm to police headquarters, deadbolts on all the doors, and stops so that windows could not be opened more than six inches. At night, a new vapor light on a thirty-foot pole in the backyard illuminated the dark hillside behind the house. I hoped all this effort would ease her fright.

Another idea popped into my head. "Mom, please consider this suggestion," I asked, fingers crossed. "How about a small dog? A puppy would be good company and also warn off anyone that comes around."

"No. No-no-no-no. I have to learn to stay by myself." This determined-to-cope-attitude came from the helpless woman who could not write a check to a utility company. Go figure.

ONE CRUCIAL PROBLEM REMAINED. UNSOLVED. Unsolvable. How were Gracie and I going to handle Mom's spells? She would act normal for months, speaking at a normal pace without monopolizing conversations or going on spending sprees or backing her car into things, but then her tempo would speed up. No one could be more fun than Mom at the beginning of one of her flights of fancy. She sometimes soared into exuberant but controllable orbits; other times she soared out of sight—without an airplane. Unfortunately, some of those flights ended in crash landings leaving relationships with friends and family members strained or shattered.

During the next few days I could tell Mom's wheels were starting to spin faster. All the signs were there:

"Diane, Kantor's is having a sale. Let's go," she said.

"I'm really not in the mood for shopping. You go ahead."

She came home with scads of new clothes. "Come see what I bought," Mom said as she emptied five shopping bags onto her four-poster bed. "Isn't this yellow dress darling? I love it. And this turquoise top? Feel this silk suit. So soft. It feels heavenly. And this raincoat was half-price. I hope this top matches my turquoise pants. Look how pretty these heels are."

Obviously there would be no sack cloth or widow's duds on Mom.

As she started hanging up her new clothes she said, "Come on, let's drive over to Wayside for dinner tonight. We'll get some of my friends, maybe

Jessie and Annie, to come too. Everybody is talking about a new restaurant. Lugio's. Luweegio's. Something like that."

"Let's do that next visit. I really need to find the rest of the information the lawyer requested before I go back."

BANG. BANG. CLUNK.

"Mom, is that you?"

"Yes, go back to sleep."

"What are you doing awake? It's four o'clock."

"Cleaning out the sewing cabinet. Sorry I woke you up. Go back to sleep. I'll be quieter."

Chitter-chatter. Gossip. Talk, talk, talk. Mom seemed to barely pause for breath from the time she awakened until she finally went to bed. My ears got tired. I wanted to scream shut up, shut up, SHUT UP. But after years of silence, of never confronting her, it was my mouth that stayed shut.

I called Gracie, hoping she could think of any practical action. "What can I do? Mom's getting worse. She's hyper. Acting frantic. Shopping. And I have yet to see her cry about Dad."

Gracie, quiet for a moment, replied, "I don't know. I've been praying about it."

"God better hurry up," I retorted, "Mom's prayed for God to make her well all her life and I haven't seen any miracles yet. We need something now."

"Diane, I don't know what you should do. She won't go see any doctors or take any medication. I'll try to think of something. Call me if she gets any worse."

I sat down. Despair washed over me. What were we going to do?

Years before, Gracie and I had felt guilty after discussing the what-ifs of Dad dying first, but decided Mom was much more likely to predecease him in a galactic auto crash. Our chilling reality—she survived him. We were going to have to take care of her. But how? That big unanswered question haunted me. I started holding frustrated conversations with Dad, asking him why he left us to manage Mom's problem and what we should do about it. Of course, he didn't answer. Or did he?

The next morning, two days before I planned to leave, Mom and I were finishing our morning coffee at the breakfast table when she reached out and picked up Dad's heavy, ornate silver napkin ring. It was an antique they had acquired early in their marriage on a trip to Fredericksburg, Virginia. I sucked in air as I watched her pull his napkin out of the ring and unfold it across her lap.

Grief, as violent and intense as a Texas thunderstorm, washed down my body. Only three weeks before, this very napkin had spread across Dad's lap during his last meal—ever. As she patted it, she looked up at me. Tears started to spill down my cheeks, but she remained dry-eyed. I still had not seen her cry. I grabbed a tissue.

The enormous reality of what has happened has to hit her soon. Will she crumble while I'm still here? Or later? What will she do? Who will help her? Grief, mingled with helplessness racked my heart and body.

Then she said the last thing I ever expected to hear.

"Diane, I want you to meet the cutest little psychiatrist I met a few weeks ago. He's young and darling. Just darling. Name's Will. Will Fisher. And I'm concerned. You know I had a little depression a few years ago and I'm afraid with Edward's changing worlds that I might have one again."

I starred at her, dumbfounded. Feeling suspended above a glass floor of hope that could shatter with the wrong response, I searched for the right words before speaking. "You're right. It could happen. It would be so smart for you to have someone like him for backup. Just in case. Do you think you can get an appointment? I'd like to meet him before I go back."

I held my breath until she reached for the phone.

My mind buzzed as I listened to her making the appointment. Where had this idea come from? Could he help?

"Good, he's going to see us this afternoon at two o'clock. Now I want you to spiff up. Get rid of that natural look. You look positively dead with no lipstick."

That afternoon as she came down the hallway toward the garage Mom looked me up and down before dictating, "Go change to a skirt. The navy one. And hurry up. We don't want to be late."

I turned and headed to the guest room to change. I slipped out of my tan slacks in a hurry, but as I zipped up my navy skirt I stopped and stared at my reflection in the vanity mirror. Thirty-six years old and I'm still jumping through hoops when she critiques how I look. Shaking my

Unexpected Help   23

head I reprimanded myself. Still a wimp. One day you will stand up to her—but not now.

I drove, aware that Mom's lack of inhibitions about being seen entering the State Mental Hospital constituted a major sign of how far beyond the normal edge she was. Living her life concerned about what people would say meant she normally would never set foot in a mental hospital for any reason, especially since some in town would recall she had a nervous breakdown when I was a child.

As I navigated the broad sunny streets, words spewed out of Mom's mouth like a water sprinkler, landing on first one topic and then another. "Did I tell you about what happened to Lucille? Somebody started calling her at all hours and hanging up. Scared her to death. Can you imagine? Oh look," she demanded, pointing out her window, "there's Jack." Honk at him. He and Fran bought the Ritter house. She's redoing everything. Inside and out. All shades of roses. Can't see Jack in a pink bed . . ."

I tuned her out, focusing on the upcoming appointment, wishing, hoping, praying Dr. Fisher could help her. What if he tries to give her pills? What should I tell him? Mom's longtime emphatic stance on no medications had been set in steel-reinforced concrete after her nervous breakdown back in the 1940s. Now, in the 1970s Thorazine pills were still the only known remedy for hyper behavior. They made her groggy and dizzy—and very determined not to take them.

As I turned the car into the parking lot at the mental hospital, Mom dictated, "Park over there in the shade. You know I can't stand to get into a hot car. Aren't the grounds pretty? Did you put lipstick on?"

Hopping out of the car, Chatty Mom set off at a rapid trot toward the red-brick colonial-style building. Then I watched her come to an abrupt stop, take a deep breath, square her shoulders and proceed at a slow, deliberate pace, head held regally. I caught up with her just as she entered the cool, spacious institutional-green hallway. She approached the receptionist who smiled and handed her a form. Mom stared at her a moment, then slapped the paper down on the counter, firmly informing her, "I'm not here as a patient. I'm a friend of Dr. Fisher and I want him to meet Diane." Startled, the receptionist looked at me and raised her eyebrows. I smiled and nodded, not wanting any paperwork to jeopardize this chance to get help. She gave me a knowing nod and explained how to get to his office. I ascended the stairs next to a totally composed genteel Southern Lady who looked just like my hyper mother. After chattering incessantly for days, Mom uttered not a single word as she sashayed her way into the doctor's office.

"Hello, Will," Mom said in a slow and calm voice. "I want you to meet my daughter Diane."

Dr. Fisher appeared about my height, five feet, eight inches. While not a big man, he had a trim athlete's build and a firm handshake. A congenial aura about him reinforced the friendly gaze from his dark brown eyes. Pleasantries were exchanged as we took seats in his sparsely furnished pale-green office with large picture windows that overlooked manicured grounds.

"To what do I owe this visit Dixie?" he asked.

Dr. Fisher and I waited.

Mom repositioned her purse on her lap, shifted her legs and glanced around the room before replying, "I wanted Diane to meet you." She hesitated before continuing, "And as you know, my husband Edward changed worlds recently, and I just wanted to know if I can call on you if I need any help in the weeks to come."

"Of course. You're going through a major life-change. I'll be happy to help in any way I can. Is there anything specific you're concerned about?"

We waited several more moments for her answer.

Looking down, she said, "About two years ago I had a little problem—a depression. Not bad. But I'm concerned that under the circumstances, it might happen again. May I call you if I start to feel a little down?" Mom glanced at him from the downward tilt of her head—a shy, demure, helpless look.

"Absolutely. It's very natural to experience some depression when a loved one passes away. Here's my office number. Feel free to call me anytime." Smiling, she took his card, still a totally calm, unperturbed lady.

"I knew I could count on you. Wasn't the symphony wonderful?" Mom turned to me to explain that they had met at a party after the performance. They chatted a few more minutes while I sat there bewildered, memories racing through my head. What a performance I had just witnessed. Oscar level. A little depression? Not a bad one? It was so bad, so horrendous, she had not been able to even answer a simple question as to whether she preferred French or Italian dressing on her salad. Zombie Mom had existed for months. But it wasn't for that single depression in her sixty-six years of life that I needed his help. Her misleading description of her problem was unbelievable to anyone who really knew her. Dr. Fisher didn't.

On the drive home I gripped the steering wheel in anger. Why didn't I speak up? I totally blew an opportunity to get help for her. For Gracie. For me. Why am I still such a wimp? What should I do now?

Later that afternoon, after stewing over my inaction and considering various options, I launched a plan. I headed toward the garage as I called out, "I'm going over to Dad's office to copy some more papers. I'll be back about five o'clock."

Seated at Dad's desk, in Dad's chair, I rubbed my hands over the smooth surface, wishing his wisdom, his calmness would rub off on me. I contemplated what I needed to do. Back and forth my self-arguments went. How can I tattle on Mom? How can I not? Is this what traitors feel like? Or is this the answer to everybody's prayers, including hers? After ten more minutes of vacillation I concluded: Gracie and I are desperate for any help and Dr. Fisher offers help—and hope.

Final decision made, I reached for the phone. The receiver slipped in my damp hand as I dialed Dr. Fisher's number.

"Hello. This is Dixie's daughter Diane. I want to thank you for seeing us so promptly today. I also need to clarify some things Mother told you. Do you have a few minutes?" Like about a month, I thought.

"Yes, I have a little time" he said. I expelled my held breath. Thank goodness he was new in town and not over-booked yet.

I launched my prepared speech, "Dr. Fisher, my mother has a severe problem but it isn't depression. She has experienced only one depressive spell, ever, but it is what she did not tell you that I think you need to know in order to help her."

I didn't go into detail with Dr. Fisher about Mom's scary behavior when I was a young child, but even then her problem was about as subtle as a tornado blasting through town.

3

Earliest Memories

"COAST, MOM, COAST," I SQUEALED as our car started down one of the few hills in our small town.

"Coast," urged Gracie from the back seat. Even at ages four and six we knew that coasting would save gas and help the airplanes fly and win the war.

Mom shifted the floor stick. Our blue coupe sped down the hill, hot wind whistling through the open windows. At the bottom, Mom tried to shift back into gear. Sputter. Sputter. The car shook and died. She tried to start it. Grind. Grind. Clunk.

"Darn-darn-darn-darn-darn." Mom's hands fluttered between the car key, a lever on the dash and the stick jutting up out of the floor. Her feet jumped between the three floor pedals. The car started. Then coughed. Then quit. Once more her hands and feet started pulling and pushing things. Finally our car jerked forward just in time for Mom to slam on the brakes for a red light. Our car shuddered to a halt and quit again. "What the heck?" She tried to start it again. Just as the light turned green, it started with a lurch.

Mom yelled to Gracie in the back seat, "HOLD ON. HOLD ON." Throwing her arm across me as I kneeled on the front seat next to her, we roared into a side street, turning in front of some cars. Tires squealed. Horns honked. Red light ahead. Other cars stopped. We didn't.

"HOLD ON TIGHT." Turning hard we bounced over the curb into the bakery parking lot. Mom swerved to miss a parked car, sped through the parking lot and across the side street, horn blaring. We raced into our filling station at a fast clip. I thought we were going to go through the station, but she stomped the brakes hard. The car screeched to a stop—and died.

Mom sat there, blinked, then laughed. "Whew. We made it."

Looking startled, the skinny garage owner stood up from the tire he was working on and trotted toward our car, wiping his dirty hands on a red rag.

"Hey Ed, find out what's wrong with this car. It keeps stalling."

Gracie and I climbed out of the car through a cloud of stinky tire fumes. With Mom's approval, we headed for the big red Coca Cola box sitting outside the station door. Lifting one side of the lid, we both blinked as cool air from the block of ice blasted across our hot faces. I couldn't reach the bottles yet, so Gracie grabbed one for us to share. We took turns sniffing the opened bottle and giggling as the fizz tickled our noses. Watching Ed and Mom, I took a sip and held the sweet liquid in my mouth until my tongue started to tingle. About the time we finished our drink, Ed poked his head over the hood and said, "Mrs. Dweller, cain't see a thang wrong. Lemme try and start 'er."

We never did know what was wrong with that car because it started right up.

I HEARD THE HALL CLOSET door open and the snap of the string that turned on the light. I lay perfectly still, holding in my sobs. My heart began pounding so hard I was sure Mom would hear it. The pile of wool blankets I was hiding under was stinging the welts on my legs. She had used a fly swatter this time.

The light snapped off. The door closed.

I was safe. For now.

GRACIE AND I CLUTCHED MOM'S hands as we walked into the hotel ballroom. A huge Christmas tree, taller than a clown on stilts, glittered with lights and shiny ornaments. The room was full of children and mothers I didn't know. Boys chasing each other, whooped so loud we almost didn't hear him.

"Ho. Ho. Ho."

The door burst open and there he stood. Just like his pictures, white beard and all. He started pulling gifts out of his sack and calling out names. I listened and waited so long I thought he had forgotten me. He finally said, "Is Diane Dweller here?" I approached, feeling scared. I silently held out my hand. Santa smiled and placed a small gold box in it. I ran back to Mom and quickly opened it. Inside, a silver charm bracelet jingled, just like the one he gave Gracie.

I could not figure out how Santa knew we would be at that party.

MOM LOVED DRESSING UP FOR parties. I liked watching her get ready. Standing by the side of her dark mahogany dressing table one evening, I watched every move as she smeared cold cream all over her face and neck and gently wiped it off with a smooth cloth. Dipping her finger into a small pot of gooey rouge, she placed three dots on each of her high cheek bones. Twisting her mouth first in one direction and then another, she smeared those dots in large circles, creating rosy cheeks. Checking the results in the mirror, she smeared on another dot.

A cloud appeared as she patted powder all over her face and neck. The powder ladies at the store mixed it until they got just the right color to suit her. Sometimes they had to start over.

Then with a brown pencil, Mom carefully drew eyebrow arches over each of her green eyes. Only a tiny line of eyebrows had grown back since she exploded the oven and burned them all off. Puckering her mouth, she slowly dabbed on lipstick, turning her thin lips into a full, dark red pout. Mom always blotted her lipstick on a tissue and then smiled at her reflection, looking for lipstick on her teeth.

I tried blotting, without the lipstick, and got a tongue full of yucky tissues.

Before hopping up from the vanity stool, Mom rolled and secured the back of her long dark brown hair over a soft tube filled with hair she called a "rat." The roll formed a thick semicircle across the back of her neck from ear to ear. Many of her friends wore rats in their hair too.

Carefully patting perfume behind each ear and on the lining of her collar, she finally looked at me and held the fragrance stopper out. "Smell. Isn't it heavenly?" I bent forward, sniffing, inhaling her mommy-scent.

I thought my Mom looked and smelled beautiful.

She told me, "When I received my very first paycheck as a nurse I went straight to the store and bought my first bottle of Belogia perfume. I had enough money left over to purchase a beautiful, soft white wool blanket. I was so embarrassed having to use those tacky quilts Granny made out of our old clothes."

THE WILD LOOK ON MOM'S face scared me more than Daddy's bedroom slipper in her raised hand. She wasn't pretty anymore. Deep frown lines formed between her flashing eyes. Her lips disappeared into an angry line. Frightened, I froze, then wailed as she jerked my arm, throwing my body over her knees. Knowing what was coming I screamed, "I'M SORRY. I'M SORRY. I didn't mean to spill it. I just wanted to smell it again."

"HOLD STILL. MOVE YOUR HANDS OR I'LL SPANK THEM TOO."

Sometimes I knew what I had done wrong. Sometimes I wasn't sure why Mom got so mad at me, so fast.

I HEARD MOM ON THE phone sounding all excited, "Jessie, call the Ritters and tell them to meet us on top of Lookout Mountain at seven. Annie's bringing her record player. Bring your records. And some drinks. And call the Lakes. See if they can come."

Mom piled blankets, pillows, a thermos of water, snacks and records in the car. "Get in, let's go," she called to Gracie and me. Mom drove up the mountain-side road, weaving in and out on the curves, finally reaching the open stone pavilion on the flat mountain top. We could see for miles in every direction.

On some evenings the Army Air Force pilots from the training base flew bombing runs. Our group of kids sat spellbound on the huge flat rocks along the edge of the mountain. Each plane flew in low toward the target below us—a tall white cone in the center of an enormous circle of large white rocks. We held our breaths as dark canisters, full of imagined explosives, sped whistling and whining toward the target. We cheered every fake bomb, even the misses.

"Take that, Hitler."

"Gotcha, you dirty Nazis."

As darkness crept across the sky, the twinkling lights on the towers at the oil refinery, miles away, turned into a fairyland castle. In the black sky north of town, I saw angels twinkling in space, not lighted oil drilling rigs.

As night fell, our mothers called us back and made beds for us with soft blankets on the car seats. Just as I closed my eyes Gracie and I heard a deep voice ask, "Dixie, cut a rug with me?" Struggling against sleep, we sat up to peer over the edge of the car window. "Boogie Woogie Bugle Boy" blared from the record player. Silhouetted against the lighted dance floor, I spied Mom jitterbugging with Mr. Lake who had something called 4-F. All the daddies liked to dance with our Mom.

Around and around he flung her—to one side and then another. We heard whoops of joy with everybody clapping and cheering as Mom danced faster and faster. When slow dance music started I watched some of the moms dancing together because most of the daddies were gone fighting in the war.

My daddy didn't get to come to many of Mom's mountain top parties. Sometimes we wouldn't see him for three or four days. He often left before Gracie and I woke up and came home after we were in bed. Mom fretted all the time that Daddy would have to go to the war, but somebody named Uncle Sam told him to stay home and work all the time cause most of the doctors from our town had already left to help the wounded soldiers.

The days Gracie and I didn't see Daddy were sad. We missed him.

SUNDAYS WERE DIFFERENT. NOT ONLY because Daddy stayed home while we were awake, but also because of church and Mom reading the Sunday funny papers to us in our yellow living room. Yellow was Mom's favorite color. Gracie and I would climb on either side of her, sinking into the puffy cushions on the brown sofa. She would read each picture, pointing out the funny happenings. I didn't understand most of them, but I didn't care. I just wanted to feel special next to her.

One Sunday Mom read only two comics strips before she began to squirm. She stopped reading. She started and stopped. Started and stopped.

"What happens next Mom," I said. I looked up and saw the frown lines between her eyes start to deepen, making her look angry. I felt her leg tense. She jumped up, turned and scowled at me with her scary face and eyes. I cringed. She glanced at Daddy, then hurried out of the room.

I stared after her, my chin trembling. I had ruined the funny paper time.

Daddy, sitting in his brown rocking chair, put his paper down and stared after her. A frown formed on his face too. He looked so sad. I made Daddy sad. Everything I did made somebody mad or sad.

EACH NIGHT AFTER DINNER MOM would announce, "Okay girls, it's time to do the dishes." She would drag the six foot long, low wooden bench that stood on end in the corner of the kitchen and place it in front of the kitchen sink. She had Granddaddy make it so Gracie, now age seven, and I, now five, could do the dishes every night. Too short to reach the counter without it, Gracie

Earliest Memories

stood on it and washed. I dried and put things away by crawling up on the wooden counter top. We were learning Responsibilities. We actually had fun doing dishes together. Gracie taught me how to blow bubble gum bubbles and how to whistle while we did the dishes.

My weekly Responsibilities included coloring the big block of white hard stuff we ate during the war in place of butter. Mom dumped the lump in a large glass bowl, tore open the packet of orange powder and sprinkled it over the white block. On my knees on a kitchen chair, I leaned over the bowl on the table. Using a wooden spoon, I tried to stir and mix the powder evenly into the hard white block. I pressed down. I mashed and stirred until my arms felt shaky. It looked all streaked and lumpy, not like butter.

"AREN'T YOU DONE YET?" Mom's angry voice asked.

Fear stabbed me. I darted a glance at her. Her mouth turned down, frightening me. I couldn't answer, words stuck and wouldn't come out.

"Let me have it. Why can't you do anything right?" She grabbed the bowl off the table. I turned, jumped down and ran, scooting under my bed as fast as I could, feeling like I could never do anything right for her.

Later that day Mom left to work with the volunteers at the Red Cross. I felt free when she went somewhere as the leader of her garden clubs and bridge clubs and church groups. Her busy days meant we girls could play without fear under the care of Alice, our part-time nanny and housekeeper. She lived in the one-room space attached to the storeroom behind our small five-room home.

About as wide as she was tall, Alice had an even larger laugh. I knew we were expected to mind her when Mom went somewhere. That was easy. Alice sang and laughed and hugged.

One day while I sat at the red Formica table in our bright yellow kitchen helping Alice snap beans, Mom turned from the sink and said, "Alice, I don't like the way you complain about some of the work, especially cleaning the pin feathers from the chickens. We won't be needing your help here anymore. You are to move by Friday."

I heard Alice suck in a breath before saying, "Yes Ma'am."

"NO. MOM, NO."

"This isn't your business Diane."

"Mom, please don't send Alice away." I jumped up and ran to hug Alice, burying my face in her bosom, tears falling fast. "Don't leave Alice. Stay here."

I turned to beg Mom not to do this and saw the anger twisting her face into Scary Mom.

"Alice, you heard me. By Friday."

"Yes Ma'am."

Only after Mom swept out of the room did I look up and see the tears sliding down Alice's dark cheeks too.

"Hush baby," she said as she reached out and wiped my wet cheek. "Tears don't do no good now."

Mom's reason for firing Alice didn't seem good enough to me. I finally settled on the real reason: It was my fault. She knew I liked Alice better than her. I decided if I liked another nanny I wouldn't show it, because then she would have to leave too.

All the hugs left with Alice.

ONE SUNNY AFTERNOON GRACIE AND I were playing dolls on the side porch when we heard screams coming from the living room. Scared, we looked at each other in alarm and headed inside to discover what caused the commotion. We came to a fast stop in the doorway. Mom and Aunt Joyce were jumping up and down and screaming, tears running down their cheeks.

"It's over. Thank God it's over."

Aunt Joyce swung me up high, whooping again and again, "It's over. It's over. My George is coming home. Thank you Lord. This horrible war is finally over."

Church bells and car horns started ringing and honking in the distance.

"Come on girls, let's go downtown," Mom said. We grabbed small American flags out of the vase on the bookshelf, piled into Mom's blue coupe and raced through the streets, cheering and waving our flags. It looked like the whole town was there. We joined the parade of honking cars driving up and down Main Street and around the courthouse square, again and again. People were dancing in the street and hugging, making this celebration better than the Fourth of July and one of Mom's big parties put together.

EACH SUMMER GRACIE AND I looked forward to a trip to Granny's farm. Mom didn't scream at us in front of other people. And she never spanked us at Granny's. I loved going there. I felt safe. Free of fear.

After a two-day sticky-hot drive across the state of Texas and part of Arkansas, we would arrive. "Honk, Daddy, HONK," Gracie and I begged, peering over the front seat as we turned into the curved drive lined with huge oak trees. HONK. HONK. Out would come our tiny Granny, wiping her hands on her apron as she hustled down the steps. She would be trying to tuck in the grey hair that had escaped from her bun. She didn't wear makeup like Mom, but I thought she looked wonderful, even when her hair got loose again. She always greeted us with big hugs and "My how you've grown."

Gracie and I considered their cotton farm as an adventure. We raced to check out everything—the white farm house sitting up on red brick pilings, the huge vegetable garden with the funny scarecrow, the latest squealing piglets and the tire swing in the towering oak tree in the back yard. But we came to an abrupt halt at the edge of the chicken yard across from the gray weathered outhouse.

There HE strutted. Each time we needed to potty, he came squawking and flying at us, trying to peck our legs. I would wait until I just couldn't. Then I would run as fast as my legs could take me toward that dark, dreadful, stinky outhouse, slamming the door in his screeching face. Inside, shaking but safe from the beaked terror, all I had to be scared of now were the creepy daddy-longlegs spiders clinging to the walls and the monsters lurking beneath the seat holes, waiting to grab me. I didn't go to the potty very often.

We didn't see Grandpa until supper time when he came in from the cotton fields. He was real tall and real thin and real quiet and always smelled like cigarette smoke. I rarely heard him say much, but he sure could beat me at checkers. Every time.

TYPICALLY, ON THE FIRST NIGHT of our visit, Granny would serve a delicious dinner of fried chicken, fresh crowder peas with pickle relish, new potatoes in hot butter and big Granny biscuits, all raised, churned and cooked right there on the farm. Granny's kitchen wasn't like ours at home. It had a huge black wood-burning stove, but no faucet or sink. To get hot water, I watched my tiny Granny lift a big heavy wooden bucket at the well on the back porch and pour water into a metal bucket that she then lugged into the kitchen to put on the hot stove. She had to haul up and heat all the water for dish washing, cooking and our twice-a-week baths in a round tin tub.

At dusk, the adults would settle into the rocking chairs on the wide porch that stretched around two sides of the house. They chatted while Gracie and I darted among the towering oak trees, capturing fireflies. Cupping our hands to keep them from flying off, we watched the miracle of those tiny little bugs blinking on and off. How did they do that?

Exhausted and sleepy at last, we would sink into a deep feather mattress, made by Granny, pull up one of Granny's quilts and fall asleep under the soft glow of a coal oil lamp.

Mom grew up on this small forty-acre cotton patch, one of six children. I didn't think about how hard it must have been growing up there—no heating or air conditioning, no bathtub or running water, no toilet, no money and only two new homemade dresses each year. She told us how poor they were and that's why she went to school to become a nurse before she married my daddy.

BACK HOME FROM GRANNY'S, I heard Mom ask Gracie from the doorway to our bedroom, "Where is Diane? Is she hiding under her bed again?" Her voice sounded cross. "What's wrong with that child?"

Looking under my bed, knowing her little sister was hiding under her bed this time, Gracie answered truthfully, "I don't see her." Gracie protected me when she could.

We shared a bedroom so small it was hard to fit a card table between our twin beds. The walls were painted blue. White trim surrounded two large windows that overlooked the shady side porch where we often played with our dolls. The hardwood floor had a small white rug between our blond wooden beds that were covered with blue bedspreads that had bumps all over them. Our beds had blue and white striped dust ruffles that made my hiding place feel safe and dark.

We each had one baby doll. Mine was named Mary. Gracie's was Betty. During the times when Mom was in her laughing mood, Mary and I often played under my bed. Bitsy would crawl under too, curling up her warm little body next to mine for a nap. Mary, Bitsy and I spent hours living in a make-believe world under that bed, me pretending to be a fairytale princess with beautiful long hair like Rapunzel. Sometimes I became Cinderella at the ball dancing with the prince. In my fantasy world a handsome prince always came and rescued me from Scary Mom.

Lying there, I often counted the six wooden slats keeping the mattress in place. That was sometimes the number of times Mom hit me during a spanking. I knew that because Gracie taught me how to count. Gracie taught me lots of things. The time seemed to drag until she came home from school. I had to spend those hours alone with Mom. Gracie became my only playmate because our small house was in a neighborhood full of old people who didn't have children.

GRACIE KNEW HOW TO KEEP from making Scary Mom mad, except for one time. I heard Mom screaming at her. Saw her grab the hair brush, throw Gracie over her knees and start whipping her. Gracie screamed with the first blow. I stood there. I couldn't move. I couldn't breathe as I watched Mom whipping my sweet sister. Rage roared through me.

A voice in my head said, "Stop her. Grab the brush and hit Mom." I tried to scream at Mom to stop, but when my mouth opened only sobs came out. "Throw yourself at Mom, grab her arm. Stop her," the voice demanded. But all I did was stand there, crying as hard as Gracie.

Shame flooded through me, making my face feel hot. Shame, not because I wanted to hit Mom, but because I didn't stop her from hitting Gracie. I didn't help Gracie.

AFTER DAD AND GRACIE LEFT the next morning Mom headed for her bedroom to get dressed. I picked up my doll Mary and decided to play where Mom wasn't—in my favorite hiding spot under the dining table where the long tablecloth hid me. Bitsy, our little dog, came too. Just as we got settled, I heard Mom's footsteps in the kitchen. Bitsy's ears perked up. I put my hand on her head, gently holding her down.

Louder steps. She's coming this way. Can I escape?

Too late. I freeze. I can't breathe. I gasp for air.

Did she hear me?

I see Mom's white high heels coming through the doorway. They're coming toward my hiding place. I try to breathe quieter through my mouth. *Too loud.*

The shoes stop next to the table.

I stop breathing.

"Diane! WHERE ARE YOU? ARE YOU UNDER THE TABLE?"

I couldn't speak. I crossed my fingers and silently repeated: Don't find me. Don't find me. This wish worked sometimes. But not this time.

She yanked up the tablecloth, "COME OUT HERE RIGHT NOW. It is nine o'clock and we have to get to your dental appointment. LOOK AT YOU. NOT READY. What am I going to do with you? You worry me to death. Go brush your hair. And put on your sandals. We need to hurry. DON'T MAKE US LATE."

I crawled out on the other side of the table and ran to my room. I wanted to keep running. Running somewhere that would be safe from Scary Mom.

MOM WASN'T ALWAYS SCARY. IN her busy-happy mood she loved to buy us clothes and get us all dressed up to go somewhere. If an event happened in our town, we were there. She took us to circuses and flower show exhibits and to see plays and music shows. I loved it when the lights dimmed in the huge auditorium and the magic started. Drum rolls rumbled from the orchestra pit, cymbals clashed and then the curtains parted, taking me into a beautiful make-believe land. Mom didn't have to tell me to sit still. I was spellbound. My favorite performances were ballets. Back at home, Gracie and I tried standing on our toes and gracefully moving our arms. It was harder than it looked.

I DIDN'T DO THINGS ON purpose to make Mom mad. I tried to be good like Gracie, to do only what Mom expected of me. As hard as I tried, I kept failing, like the time I knocked over my glass of milk and she exploded in a fit of rage and whipped me.

During the weeks Scary Mom didn't go away, I got real good at disappearing. Keeping out of Mom's sight might have been a fun game like hide-and-seek if I hadn't been so scared all the time. So afraid of her. I don't remember when I first got scared. There would be some long times when Mom was fun and I almost forgot to be afraid of her. But they didn't last. Scary Mom always came back.

4

Frantic Survival

MOM CALLED FOR GRACIE AND me to come into her peach-colored bedroom with the pretty roses in the rug. "I have something special to show you." She smiled as she opened a drawer in her antique mahogany dresser and lifted out a tissue-wrapped bundle. She carried it to her high four-poster bed and carefully opened it. Inside, we saw a tiny white knitted sweater and cap and several little blue gowns that would fit our dolls.

"These are clothes for the new baby who is coming to live with us," Mom said.

"A baby? When?" Gracie and I grinned and started jumping up and down.

"Soon."

"Can we take care of her?"

"You can help. We are hoping to have a baby boy this time," Mom said smiling.

"Where do you get babies?" Gracie asked.

Mom opened her mouth, closed it, paused, then said, "At the hospital. Grandmother Dweller will come and take care of you while I go to the hospital to get our new baby. Daddy and I have prayed for five years for this baby and now we're going to get him."

We got our dolls Mary and Betty and all their clothes and our favorite, colorful, doll-sized quilts Grandmother Dweller had made just for us. We played "new baby brother," rocking, diapering and feeding our baby dolls over and over.

One morning when we woke up, Grandmother was making coffee in the kitchen. "Where's Mom?" we asked.

Grandmother's eyes got all teary as she said, "Children, come here. Your mom and dad are at the hospital." She sat down on a kitchen chair and reached out her arms to us.

"Did they get the new baby yet? Did they get our brother?"

"Sweethearts, it is hard to understand, but sometimes things are not meant to be. We don't know why, but something went wrong and your mother won't be coming home with a baby after all."

"Why not? If something went wrong with this baby, why don't they ask the hospital for another one?" Gracie asked.

Later our parents took us out to the cemetery to show us where our baby sister was sleeping in the ground. That's when I knew for sure that we weren't going to get another baby.

A WEEK LATER GRACIE STARTED tossing everything out of the bottom of our small closet while I searched under our beds and then out on the side porch.

"Mom, we've looked everywhere for our doll quilts. We can't find them."

"I threw them away."

Gracie stared at Mom. Her bottom lip started to tremble, "Why, Mom, why? Grandmother made them for our dolls. We love them."

"Only poor people use quilts," she declared. "You don't want those quilts."

Yes we did.

AFTER OUR BABY DIDN'T COME home Mom stayed busy, busy, busy, always in a hurry. Always angry.

"Don't bother me."

"Clean this up right now."

"You girls, you girls, I don't know what I am going to do with you."

"YOU KNOW BETTER THAN THAT."

"TURN OVER RIGHT NOW." Her face would get red and scary. She would grab me, throw me over her knees and start hitting. Whack. I would feel her hairbrush hit. Again. And again.

In the months after our baby died Mom's actions became even scarier. She didn't sleep. She woke us up banging pots in the kitchen late at night. She fretted and yelled, telling us what everyone had to do—or else. Nothing I did pleased her. Scary Mom didn't go away. Her constant screaming created teeth-grinding fear in me, making my jaw hurt. I stayed scared of her, always wondering what would set her off, never sure what action—or inaction—would result in a whipping. Without a warning when something made her mad, she would scream at me, snatch up Dad's long-handled wooden clothes brush—or whatever item she could grab first—shoes, hair brushes, fly swatters—grab me, throw me over her lap, and start hitting.

"I'M SORRY, I'M SORRY. DON'T HIT ME," I wailed each time. That never stopped her.

Sometimes during a whipping she screamed at me, "IF YOU DON'T STOP SCREAMING I'LL SPANK YOU UNTIL YOU DO." I would try to stop crying. That's hard to do when she is hitting and hitting until her arm gets tired.

Scary Mom only used one way to punish me, no matter what I did. No time outs. No taking away my favorite toys or books. No explanation of what I did wrong before or after her dreaded spankings. When she let go of me, I would run and hide under my bed or the dining table, sobbing.

EACH NIGHT WHEN I CRAWLED in bed, after turning the top of the sheet neatly over the blue bedspread, I pressed my palms together to say my prayers. "God, please make Mom go away so I can live with just Daddy. Please. That is all I want. In Jesus name. Amen."

When God didn't make Mom go away and she kept screaming and spanking me I became desperate. I had to get away from her. I knew I had to run away. Where could I go? How would I get there? I needed to figure out how.

I sat cross-legged on my bed and shook my piggy bank until all my money fell out. Gathering up the nickels, dimes and pennies, I counted them and thought through my plan. I knew how to get on the city bus to get to the big bus station. But then where? All our relatives lived far, far away. I tried to figure out what to do, but could not come up with a safe place to go, or more money. The thought of going off by myself made me so scared I felt cold all over. Gracie came into our bedroom about this time, her thick auburn hair in damp curls, a jump-rope in her hand. "What are you doing?" she asked, looking at my small pile of money.

"Gracie, Mom's mad all the time. I'm scared of her." I started sobbing. "I'm going to run away. Come with me. Maybe we can go to Dallas. Please. Please."

She stared at me a moment, then sat down on the bed next to me looking sad too. "I know. But you can't run away. You're too little. I'm too little. We can't do that. The police will bring us back." Her shoulders slumped. Mine slumped too. I felt stuck. Trapped. Then I declared, "I may be too little to leave now, but when I'm ten, I'm leaving."

DAY AFTER DAY MY FEAR of making Scary Mom mad increased. Bewildered, frightened, I kept watching, hiding, praying. All I could think about was how to get away from her.

When I opened my eyes each morning I went on alert. Where is she? I would listen carefully for any sound, knowing Daddy and Gracie had already gone to work and school. As soon as I heard her, usually in the kitchen, my stomach would start hurting.

I may have been a slow learner about what not to do, but I did learn it was best to stay out of Scary Mom's sight, to vanish until I had to show up for lunch. On cold days or when the sand was blowing I would have to hide from her in the house, listening always for her footsteps. When I heard her coming, I would tiptoe the other way, my heart beating fast. Stop. Listen. Where is she going next? I became afraid of getting trapped in rooms that had only one door. The kitchen, dining room and living room all had two doors I could use to escape.

Then one night Mom's upset voice woke me up. "NO, NO, NO. I'm not crazy. I'm NOT going to a mental hospital. I'm not sick. What is wrong with helping others? If I don't help them, who will? I'm praying for God's help."

I could barely hear Daddy's quiet voice. "Dixie, we're going ... see what ... help ..."

"Don't take me to a mental hospital. WHAT IF THEY LOCK ME UP? OR DO SHOCK TREATMENTS? YOU CAN'T TAKE ME THERE. I'LL SLOW DOWN. I'll rest more," I heard Mom break into sobs. "Don't you love me?"

"I do love you. We're just going to the clinic. And I won't let them lock you up. For the sake of our marriage and the girls, we have to get some help for you."

So, when I was six, Daddy took Mom to Galveston to his medical school to see the doctors there. At church the next Sunday I overheard adults whispering words like "crazy" and "nervous breakdown" and "poor little girls."

Did God answer my prayers? Was Mom going away and not coming back?

Gracie and I went to stay with an older, childless couple for the month. I loved the attention I received. And for the first time, bedtime stories were read to me. And hugs. Wonderful warm hugs. No one yelled at me, corrected me or whipped me for a whole month. Slowly, I felt tension start to leave my body, my constant upset tummy stopped churning. I started to laugh, even giggle, feeling happy. Free of fear.

I prayed hard that Mom would never come back. When asked if I missed her, I politely nodded my head 'yes' when I really wanted to say "no."

The doctors in Galveston didn't have much luck slowing Mom down. She told us what a good time she had. She got Daddy to take Arthur Murray dance lessons. "You know how I love to dance. I told him we could learn all the fancy dance steps like the tango, samba and rumba. Daddy really tried," she reported, "but the rhythm didn't reach his feet."

Mom told everyone, "The doctors say I'm fine. All I need to do is slow down and take a nap every day." Every afternoon that summer, at one o'clock, we girls had to take what Mom called a "siesta." Gracie napped with Mom on her high, four-poster bed while I stretched out on a pallet made of blankets on the floor. Wafts of musty air blew over me from the window cooler as the water dripped over straw mats, trying to cool the hot Texas air. I guess we had to take naps too so we would be quiet and Mom would know where we were. But a nap is a nap, and at six I didn't want to nap. We couldn't talk or wiggle. Some days that siesta seemed to last forever.

In the weeks after their return Mom seemed happier, not so angry. In fact, our whole family seemed happier. While Daddy still worked long days, he was home more, especially at night for dinner. Each night Gracie and I set the table while Mom cooked. Sometimes she made fried chicken, our favorite. We four would sit down to a hot dinner and bow our heads for Daddy to say the blessing. Sometimes he asked Gracie or me to say one.

It was not unusual for our meals to be interrupted by the phone ringing. Mom would jump up and go to the phone shelf in the hall to answer it. Often she would call out, "Edward, it's the hospital calling." He would disappear into the hall and we could hear him asking questions and then saying, "I'll be right down."

Mom would kiss him goodbye as he went out the door. Turning back to the table, she would look sad and say, "After working all day he gets called back. Over and over. And he's so tired."

MOM'S FRANTIC BEHAVIOR SLOWED DOWN after Daddy and the doctors made her stop going to every club but one. She chose one of her garden clubs—plus church. But it wasn't long before she headed the Sunday School Program and started visiting church newcomers and going to see sick and old people. She sure could fill up a day with church doings.

Sometimes Mom had to take big pills to calm down. She would pout and beg Daddy not to make her. "I'll slow down. I promise. No more of those awful pills. Please. They make me feel awful."

She would try, really try to calm down for a day or two, but then he would get out the pills. They made her sleepy and talk really slow, like Mom's friend from Alabama.

Mom's siesta, plus those pills, did help her slow down, but she still got real angry during what Gracie started calling "spells." They lasted for weeks and I dreaded them. Busy Mom always lived with us, but Super-Busy-Screaming-Scary Mom showed up during those spells.

While angry whippings still occurred after the Galveston trip, most angry corrections came now, not with Dad's shoe or hairbrush, but with words. Over and over I heard, "Why can't you do anything right?" I decided the saying, "Sticks and stones may break your bones but words can never hurt you," was wrong. Mom's spankings hurt my bottom. Her words hurt my head. And my heart.

I disappeared as much as possible. I promised myself that someday I would disappear from her for good.

MOM'S RELIGION PLAYED A BIG part in her life, and in ours. Weekly we attended the Sunday morning services at the First Baptist Church, evening bible study classes and preaching services, plus Wednesday night prayer meetings. One Sunday morning we had a special speaker. He had flown his private plane to North Creek for the occasion and planned to fly the fifty miles to the next town that afternoon to speak at a church there.

I could feel Mom's excitement as she approached him after the service.

Frantic Survival 43

With a flirty smile and twinkle in her eye, she inquired in her party voice, "Would you have room in your plane for a lady who just wants to fly? I've never flown and I would love for you to show me all about it." Within the hour, Dad, Gracie and I were riding down the highway to pick her up in the next town, searching the sky to catch a glimpse of our mother flying over us.

Our Mom sure did some exciting things.

How pretty we looked ranked high on Mom's checklist, right next to how well we behaved. Our shoes were always shined and our hair always curled—or frizzed. Her daily correction about my appearance made me aware that looking pretty was very important to her.

Mom often expressed frustrations with my thin, limp hair. Weekly, she would pin-curl it after my shampoo, creating curls that would last a few hours. Then one week, after washing my hair at the kitchen sink, she said, "Diane, you can set your own hair now." She stacked Daddy's brown footstool on top of her peach-colored stool so I could see in her vanity mirror. I climbed up both stools.

"Gracie, come help me out in the yard. We need to get that flat of petunias in the ground."

They left me sitting there, staring wide-eyed at my reflection, watching the water drip off the ends of my hair. Panic threatened. I had watched Mom making pin-curls, but had never, ever, tried it myself.

How did she do it? What if I didn't do it right?

With unsure hands, I took a clump of my short hair and tried to make a circle of it against my head with my right hand. Stretching carefully to grab a bobbie pin off the top of the vanity, I almost fell. Lost the curl. Tried again. Finally sliding off both stools, I grabbed a bobbie pin, climbed back up both stools and made another curl. Only my fingers could not open the bobbie pin with only one hand. I let go of the curl, opened the pin and stuck it on my first finger. Then I make another curl. Getting the pins off my finger and onto the curls became harder and harder as my hair got drier and drier. I struggled and struggled and finally had four pinned curls, all in stages of uncurling.

Tears of frustration dripped off my chin as I sat there, awaiting my punishment, knowing what Mom would do when she discovered my failure.

As I heard her footsteps in the hall coming my way, I grabbed the edges of the stool to keep my hands from shaking. Mom looked really mad when she saw my hair, but she must have realized she had asked me to do something that was too hard. She took over in silence, her mouth in a straight line. I had failed again to do anything right, but at least she didn't whip me this time. She took me to the beauty shop to get my first permanent. She said it would make my hair curly.

The beauty operator set me on cushions in her chair and rolled up a machine that looked like a huge helmet with lots of thick electrical wires dangling down like octopus legs. Each wire had a metal clamp on the end. The operator coiled wet strands of my hair around a curler, then fastened the curler to one of the dangling clamps.

As she worked her way around my head clamping more and more curlers to the machine, I stayed as still as I could. Tiring, I tilted my head down. "OUCH," I yelped as the clamps all over my head pulled my hair. My scalp was still hurting when she announced, "Now don't move or you'll get burned." Soon after she flipped the "On" switch I started to feel heat all over my head. Then a clamp started burning my scalp. I jerked my head, trying to pull away from the pain only to cry out as more strands of hair were yanked and other spots started to burn. This torture lasted forever.

Maybe, just maybe, if I ever had bouncy, soft curls like Shirley Temple it might have been worth it, but not even hot waves could thicken my thin, fine brown hair. I would end up with nothing to show for the torture but the frizzes. I couldn't sing or dance like Shirley either.

Mom did try to introduce us to music. A moving van delivered a dark mahogany upright piano with a mirror attached to the front. Clapping with excitement, I couldn't wait for my first lesson.

I sat on the bench next to my teacher and tried to understand what she told me. Week after week I tried to follow her directions. While I could read a few words in books, reading music made no sense to me. My tone-deaf ears couldn't connect the notes, the keys and the sounds together, nor could my fingers find the right keys, like Gracie's. Unable to make the piano sound like the teacher wanted, my excitement quickly died. Each lesson meant I failed again. A year later Mom switched me to another teacher. The problem wasn't the teacher.

At least while practicing my scales I did have fun making weird faces in that mirror.

Each piano lesson day I begged, "Please let me stop piano and take art lessons." Constantly drawing everything on anything, I seldom went anywhere without my colored pencils. By age seven my weekly visits to the library found me in the research section, looking for books on theater costumes to bring home. Hours disappeared as I drew, designed and cut out colorful costumes for my paper dolls.

Mom ignored my drawing. "You are absolutely not stopping piano. You-are-going-to-learn-to-play-the-piano. Sit-down-there-and-practice."

The one lesson I did learn was that if I started practicing right after lunch, Mom would ask me to stop so she could take her daily nap. Finally she realized how useless it was to continue my piano lessons. But my excitement over the end of the piano-torture evaporated when she declared, "We've spent all this money on piano lessons and we're not going to waste money on art lessons."

Mom did like to spend money on clothes though.

Party Mom loved pretty clothes, not only for herself but for us too. She reminded us Granny made her only two new school dresses each year. Her too-small last year's dresses were worn during the long hours she hoed weeds in the hot, humid fields of their cotton farm. Now she could have lots of pretty clothes, and so could we. Off we would go in Mom's car, speeding down the broad streets to The Kid's Shop. The faces of the salesladies brightened when they saw us walk in the door. Clothes were selected from the racks; more brought to the dressing room; complete outfits were suggested. We would leave with boxes and bags of beautiful new school and play clothes and special Sunday church clothes—fancy dresses, ruffled petticoats, lacy socks, shiny patent leather Mary Jane shoes, straw hats and white gloves.

One fall shopping trip Mom spied a white rabbit fur coat and muff in my size. She was ecstatic, "Oh look. How adorable. A fur coat. My daughter will have a real fur coat. I wish you had one in my size," she said, rubbing her hand over the soft fur. I wore that coat until my arms stuck out of it like Popsicle sticks.

FINALLY, I WENT TO SCHOOL too. I loved it. My really tall teacher was strict and frowned a lot, but she didn't scream at us or spank anyone. I made good grades and wanted to go to school every day, even during Christmas holidays. I felt safer there.

Each day, after my school day ended, I joined six other first-graders to play in the school yard while waiting the half hour for our big brothers and sisters to get out of the higher grades and our mothers to come pick us up.

"Girls chase the boys," we girls yelled. I headed for cute Jerry with the black hair and dark eyes. He dashed across the bare, rocky playground with me running fast behind him. Over the curb we went, across the dirt side street and pell-mell down the steep hillside. Slip, slide. My feet flew out from under me. I fell forward and felt a stabbing, sharp pain in my leg. "AHHHAAA, AHHAAA." A broken piece of glass was sticking out of my knee. Blood started pouring from the wound and running down my leg. Everybody started screaming. Soon Mrs. Parks, the school principal, stood over me. She had a big frown on her face and looked mad. The janitor picked me up and we made a bloody path back to the school office. I kept crying until Daddy arrived.

"Now let's take a look and see what we have here," his soft voice calmed me. I sucked in air, trying to be brave, while he pulled pieces of glass out of my leg and pressed big bandages over the still bleeding wound.

Before we left for the hospital, two blocks away, Mrs. Parks said again and again, "I've told them many times not to play over there." That was a lie. She had never ever told us not to. Not once. Why was she telling Daddy a lie? Teachers aren't supposed to lie. Lying is a sin.

Daddy carried me into his office at the hospital, laid me on the examining table and poured something cold over my gaping cut. I could see the bones inside my knee. Feeling sick and weak and cold and shaky all over, I started crying again just as Mom came bursting in the door of the room. "What happened? Oh God. What happened?"

I raised my arms out to her.

"Oh, this is awful." She took one look at my leg and turned away from me.

"Mom, Mom," I sobbed, reaching out to her. Mom, who used to be a nurse, walked out. Daddy frowned at her back a moment before turning toward me. He had to give me shots in my knee before he sewed it up. It hurt. Bad. Almost as much as Mom leaving.

Later, back home in my blue bed, feeling abandoned by Mom when I needed to be hugged, I imagined this scene: I saw Mom's car going fast down

Frantic Survival

a steep hill, flipping over, somersaulting like I had. The windows would break and she would get cut and I wouldn't hug her—ever. Or maybe, maybe she would die. Good. Then I wouldn't have to run away and I could live with just my daddy.

Revenge had entered my six-year-old soul.

DURING A SUMMER VISIT TO Granny's farm without our parents, Gracie and I begged Granny to let us climb up and explore the barn loft. With her approval, we scampered across the back yard—barely ahead of that squawking rooster—and into the weathered, gray barn. Yuck. Stinky manure. Rays of sunlight filled up with the dust moats our feet stirred up from dried corn husks. I started breathing through my mouth.

The ladder, located in a back stall, loomed taller than any I had ever seen. Gracie started up. I climbed up behind her. At the top I looked at the big gap between the ladder and the loft floor, not sure my shorter legs could make it. My knees started to wobble. I reached out to Gracie on the landing. She grabbed my arm and with a hard yank, helped me land safely.

The doors in the front of the loft were open, providing plenty of light for exploring. Looking around, we skirted the red potatoes spread across most of the loft floor where they would stay dry for some future meal. Back in the shadows we spied a humpbacked trunk. Treasures beckoned. Opening it, we were disappointed to discover just bunches of old newspapers from the 1890s, cut up into the clothing patterns. Granny had used them to sew clothes for other people to make money.

Digging deeper in the trunk, we found bound bundles of report cards for each of Granny's six children. "Let's read Mom's," Gracie said. Mom often told us what a smart student she had been, especially in math. Gracie shuffled through the cards and handed one to me. "Look Diane, she has a lot of A's and B's, but there's a C, and here's another C in the tenth grade. She didn't tell us about those." Flipping several over, Gracie saw some comments from her teachers. She read them out loud. "This one says 'Highly nervous.' Another says 'Very excitable.' And here's one that has 'Needs to settle down' on it."

We knew what that meant.

WHEN OUR PARENTS CAME TO pick us up at the end of our visit, Mom started rearranging Granny's furniture.

"Edward, Ned, come help." Mom demanded, calling to Daddy and her brother.

"Dixie, don't rearrange the furniture again," Dad said, shaking his head.

"Yes, this way isn't as good as what I have planned. Come on. Help," she said as she tugged at the sofa's arm. "Ned, you get on that end, Edward on this one. Move it over here." The two men looked at each other, shrugged their shoulders and picked up the sofa.

When Granny came into her living room, she silently eyed the new arrangement. Her smile disappeared into a straight line. But like everyone else, Granny didn't bother to protest Mom's decisions. She, too, knew it would be useless.

After we left, Granny always moved the furniture back the way she wanted it. You would think that would stop Mom on her next visit, but no, the furniture always got rearranged. Once Mom decided to take charge or change something, she could not be stopped.

MOM TOLD US THE BOOKS she read when she was a girl revealed that not everyone lived in poverty like her family did. Books. By the time I was in third grade, books showed me my mother was different. None of the mothers in the books like the *Bobbesy Twins* and *The Swiss Family Robinson* whipped or screamed at their children. After I read *Pollyanna,* about the girl who learned how to be glad in spite of her grumpy Aunt Polly, I tried to play the glad game—glad Dixie was my Mom. That lasted until Mom yelled at me about an hour later. I couldn't even be "glad" right.

Knowing what would happen if we did not behave like Mom expected us to, Gracie and I became super obedient. Once we showed her we could behave, she took us to many different events she had never experienced during her childhood. In the next few years, on family trips to Dallas and Austin, we attended operas, symphonies, the theater and ice skating shows. Mom seemed as delighted by them as we were. While I loved the theater, the excitement of performances and travel, they were just things we did, often with added feelings of stress to always be on our best behavior.

Going special places with Mom was exciting, but a hug would have thrilled me more.

Frantic Survival 49

AFTER DINNER ONE NIGHT, DADDY didn't head for his brown rocking chair in the living room to study his medical books as usual. Instead, he placed a big square board and big sheets of paper on the dining room table. Mom, still wearing her blue flowered apron, sat down next to him. Curious, I went to see what was up. Standing by the side of the table I watched every move as Daddy used what he referred to as a T-square and a triangle-shaped ruler to start drawing what Mom called a floor plan. Daddy's house plans would show an architect what they wanted in our new house.

Mom made frequent suggestions. "Make the den larger, longer. And I want a huge pantry off the kitchen. No, no. Don't put the utility room there. Move it across the hall from the kitchen." Mom kept changing her mind. Daddy, patient as usual, kept changing it on the paper.

Fascinated with how he could make rooms appear, connect and change, I wanted to do that too. The next day, I tried to make rooms fit together on some of Daddy's extra paper. It turned out to be harder than it looked. I needed a big eraser. Then I discovered some of Mom's magazines had house plans that I could trace and change.

Reading a book on the side porch a week later I looked up when the postman walked by and saw him putting some magazines in our mailbox. Hoping they were a *House Beautiful* or *Home and Gardens,* I headed out. Yes. One house magazine. Standing at the mailbox, I eagerly turned the pages until I spied a house plan. I saw instantly how to make the plan better. I would add a second doorway to all the rooms so the children could always escape.

OVER THE NEXT YEAR I watched our new house magically appear. I absorbed every detail, the pouring of the foundation, the framing of the walls, and then the roof. I couldn't wait to discover the changes every visit. Each new detail seemed like an exciting present. What fun. At age ten, I decided to become an architect when I grew up.

Finally we moved into the results of all this planning. Constructed of white Austin stone, our long, low ranch house had a contrasting dark redwood front porch and eaves. Built on a hillside, concrete retaining walls created terraces at the street level and behind the house.

Gracie and I shared a spacious bedroom on the front of the house. It had a row of chest-high windows that revealed the shallow valley that held the center of town. As soon as I awakened each morning, I kneeled on my bed to peer out those windows, "Oh drat, Gracie. Here comes the dust again. Oklahoma is going to be blowing past us by mid-morning." I could tell that by looking at the low band of grey stretched across the horizon.

Spring sandstorms became an everyday event in our town during that long drought in the 1950s. We tried sticking masking tape around all the windows. Still, the dust blew in. It got into everything, especially our drafty old school building. The sand in the air became so thick inside, we couldn't see the end of the hall. Grit covered our desks and school papers. Outside, I never stood still but either ran or jumped up and down. If I didn't keep moving the sand hit with such force it stung like sharp needles, sandblasting my legs.

A never-ending task at our new home was sweeping the sand out of the garage and off the porches, plus pulling all the weeds that had sprouted in the top soil the contractor spread across our long front yard. Week after week Gracie and I spent hours after school and on Saturdays, when the sand wasn't blowing, hand-pulling weeds with the promise of getting paid for this extra job. That was a joke on us.

"Mom, you forgot to pay us for pulling up the weeds."

"I paid you."

"That was last week Mom." Gracie and I chimed in unison.

"Are you sure?"

"Yes. We're sure. You didn't pay us," we insisted.

"I'm sure I did." This weekly scene resulted in sometimes getting paid, sometimes not. Attempts to get a regular allowance met with the same accounting problems, often leaving us broke and frustrated.

One day, walking down the hall past the kitchen I heard Daddy chide Mom in a stern voice, "Dixie, Charles called me from the bank again today. You have overdrawn your account again. I've put more money into it, but you have to keep track of your spending better."

Ha, I grinned. Mom was in trouble.

5

Mom's Spells

L IFE BEGAN TO CHANGE IN my pre-teen years. I started to doubt my early childhood belief that I was the cause of Mom's scary behavior because she continued to have spells even when I behaved. It slowly became clear to Gracie and me that Mom's periodic frantic actions followed a pattern.

Late in the spring of my first year in junior high, Gracie and I noticed the signs that another spell had started. Mom became exuberant, laughing, full of energy.

"Girls, Kantor's is having a sale. Let's go shopping."

Off we went to our favorite store. Gracie and I waded in among the crowd of bargain hunters. Looking through the racks, we chose a couple of dresses each. Mom joined us, "Oh look at this one. And that one. Try them on too." She added more and more dresses, skirts and tops to our piles. Loaded with items, Gracie and I shared a dressing room, taking turns changing into new garments and going out to show Mom. By then, she would have even more items for us to try on. We walked out of the store with shopping bags bulging with new clothes.

Getting back in the car, I thought we were going home, but Mom turned the car toward the center of town. "I need some new shoes. Let's go see what The Shoe Rack has in stock. All six of our extra narrow feet trooped into the store to the welcoming smiles of the salesladies who knew us by name. Within twenty minutes boxes upon boxes littered the floor around our chairs. A considerable number of shoes went home with us too.

"Let's go shopping," turned out to be a definite signal that another spell had started, but over the years it became harder and harder for us to get excited over new clothes. We knew what would follow.

At bedtime a few nights later, another clue surfaced. As Gracie and I completed our nighttime rituals—pin curls, freckle-erase cream and calamine lotion for blemishes, she said, "Let's go get a scoop of ice cream. I think we have some chocolate chip."

When we entered the kitchen, I noticed our back yard ablaze with lights.

"Why are all the outside lights on?" I asked.

Gracie peered out. "Mom's out there."

"What's she doing? It's almost ten o'clock." We could see Mom bending over aggressively digging in a flowerbed, dirt flying.

"Planting some flowers?" Gracie raised her eyebrows and shrugged.

When hyper, whatever Mom hankered to do, she did, regardless of the time of day, the weather, the cost or the logic.

During the initial period of fun activities, Mom planned parties, often inviting two or more couples for dinner. Gracie and I helped get everything ready and cleaned up the dishes, but preferred to eat in the breakfast room rather than attend her dinner parties.

One evening as I entered the den to clear the dishes after the guests had moved over to the bamboo lounge chairs, I heard Mom chattering away, jumping from one topic to another. Then I heard Dad chide her, "Dixie, let someone else talk."

Wow. I stood there dumbfounded. Hearing Dad correct Mom in front of others shocked me. I looked at her. She opened her mouth, then closed it. She looked chastened. But she did shut up. For a few minutes.

WHEN MOM'S ACTIVITIES INTENSIFIED, HER senses did too. "Oh smell this. Smell. It's fantastic," she said, waving a dish of peach cobbler under my nose. Or smacking her lips, she declared, "Taste this tomato soup. I have never tasted any this good before. The flavor's incredible." I smelled, I tasted, and thought whatever she seemed so ecstatic about just smelled or tasted normal. After a spell ended, she would often lament, "Things don't taste as good as they used to."

During spells, Mom's inability to sleep increased. One night we awoke to BANG, BANG, BANG about three in the morning. It was Mom, frantically slamming the iron down on some garment on the ironing board.

As soon as the sun crept up enough to lighten the sky, she began a Herculean gardening task with gusto. Any plant that refused to do her bidding by not growing big enough or flowering just right, or that just

Mom's Spells 53

looked tacky to her, found itself uprooted and flying into the garbage pile.

When Dad insisted Mom slow down, she replied, "I'm busy. I have to get this done. No. I am NOT going to take that awful pill. Don't make me. I'm praying for calm. I'll be calmer. Just let me finish this."

During a spell Mom focused on whatever was popping into her brain, not on the traffic—or pedestrians—or our safety. She typically drove too fast, but during this spell "fast" took on a new meaning. Gracie and I didn't want to get in the car with her because her driving turned out to be hair-raising scary, like the time she didn't stop for a lady in a crosswalk.

"WATCH OUT." Gracie shrieked. "Mom, you almost hit that woman. You're supposed to stop for people in crosswalks."

"She saw me."

Yeah, and ran for her life, I thought, shaking my head. I suspected that woman was shaking all over.

A couple of blocks later, Gracie yelled, "MOM, STOP."

Mom turned to look where we were headed—into an intersection. She hit the brakes hard and came to a screeching halt. The car rocked back. Traffic whizzed by inches away from our front bumper. She had been looking out her side window at someone's yard.

When the light turned green, she floor-boarded the gas pedal. Thrown back in my seat, I watched the speedometer needle spin, hitting forty-five miles an hour by the middle of the next block. As she careened around a corner, Gracie and I struggled to stay upright. I grabbed the arm rest and held on.

It's a wonder the local drag racers didn't challenge her.

"Dixie," Dad warned at dinner a few nights later, "you must slow down before you hurt someone. And be more careful backing up. Look where you are going. Our insurance rates have gone up because of your driving record." Mom looked down at her plate and nodded her head without saying a word. She may have had good intentions to slow down, but during a spell she rarely ever went the speed limit—inside or outside of the car.

One afternoon Mom drove up the slightly sloping driveway at a friend's house and the three of us piled out of the car. Mom, Gracie and I were no more than five steps away from it when Mom started screaming, "STOP. STOP. SOMEBODY STOP THE CAR."

She started running after it, frantically waving her arms. She had forgotten to put it in Park. We watched helplessly. The blue Buick picked up speed, rolled down the driveway, crossed the road, jumped the curb and crushed large shrubs before landing down in a gully. A tow truck and another lecture from Dad did nothing to make her more attentive.

When Mom put the car in reverse it was always an adventure, but none more so than when she backed out of our garage during this spell. A curve in the driveway design allowed her to back out around the curve and then pull forward into the street. This time the trouble occurred when Mom started turning the wheels *before* she cleared the garage. In her hurry-up mood, she hit the gas and started backing out fast. CRUNCH. LURCH. STOP. She had managed to hook the edge of the front bumper on the stone column between the car stalls. After the tow truck man got us unhooked and left, she asked, "Do you think Dad will notice?" The bumper, pulled several inches away from the front of the car on one side, listed at an angle.

"What happened to the car bumper?" was the first thing we heard as Dad came in from the garage that night. While many men would get mad and rant, my calm Dad just sighed, shook his head and had it repaired.

Many of Mom's reckless driving issues were due to her inattention, but some of her bad driving habits may have formed in her youth. She never had a driving lesson or driving test. When a teenager, Mom mailed twenty-five cents to the state of Arkansas; they sent back a mail-order driver's license. After she moved to Houston she exchanged that license for a Texas license that she kept renewing over the years.

As soon as Gracie passed her Texas driver's test at age fourteen she became our chauffeur, especially during Mom's spells. What a relief.

"GO GET DRESSED," MOM SAID at the breakfast table one Saturday morning, "you can come with me to the hospital and help me repot all the ivy plants there."

I dressed, combining my favorite dark blue pleated skirt with a light green blouse, navy barrettes in my hair and green socks with navy shoes on my feet. I liked the effect as I checked out my image in the full length mirror on the back of our closet door. Mom came into my room, took one look at me and frowned. "Diane, you are not leaving the house looking like that.

Blue and green are never worn together. It's tacky. No. No. No. And polish those shoes."

I clenched my teeth, wanting to scream: Why can't you ever say something nice to me? Will you ever stop criticizing me?

Over the years I learned that refusing to obey Mom's commands instantly was not a smart option, especially during a spell. But in daydreams, night dreams, and imaginary scenarios I did refuse. I became determined to tell her off, rehearsing retorts silently in my head while on my bike, in the shower, or drying the dishes. I plotted different scenarios; my mind seethed with ugly names like Witch. Witch. I grinned, imagining Mom melting into the ground like the witch in the *Wizard of Oz*, her tiny eyebrows the only thing left.

I had tried to convince myself that the next time, the very next time Mom criticized me I would yell at her: STOP CRITICIZING ME. Seething over this latest criticism of my clothes, I still hesitated to scream those words at her. Instead I marched into the closet, threw my clothes on the floor and put together another outfit I knew she wouldn't like. I came out of my room wearing a defiant smile and mismatched clothes, daring her to send me back to the closet again.

My first silent confrontation didn't work. Too impatient to wait, she had left without me.

The next day when I started to sit down for breakfast Mom spoke up, "Diane, what have you done to your hair? It looks awful. Go do it the way I showed you. Right now."

I stood there staring at her, urging myself to yell one of my well-practiced retorts back. Instead, dragging my feet, shoulders slumped, I headed down the hall to the bathroom vanity and the curlers, mumbling under my breath, "Wimp. Wimp. Wimp."

I wasn't the only one who became a target of Mom's negative comments during this spell. Stopped at a traffic light, we watched a heavyset woman start across the street in front of our car. "Isn't that disgusting? Look how fat she is. How sloppy," Mom frowned and shook her head. "I don't know why people let themselves get so fat."

Mom took care to keep her own figure trim and to always be perfectly groomed. She glowed when a compliment came her way, but her constant criticisms had trained me not to ever expect a compliment from her. Thus my goal each day became to avoid the silent stare and negative shake of her head—or to be sent back to fix my hair—or shoes—or skirt. Every day I checked out my appearance, longing for one smile, one "you look nice," or even one nod that meant I had her approval.

If you never expect a compliment—or a hug—you shouldn't be disappointed that you never get one. I kept hoping that one day, one day, a compliment or a hug—or a miracle—might happen.

DURING EVERY SPELL, INCLUDING THIS one, Mom would become increasingly insensitive to other peoples' feelings and reactions to her. Unfortunately, Mom's brother and his wife arrived from Arkansas for a visit of several days. They settled into the guest room.

Mom had scheduled a dinner party in our home for that evening, but instead of including my aunt and uncle in the party, she called them into the den where Gracie was setting the dining table.

Mom said, "We're having a dinner party tonight for some friends, but since you don't know any of the guests you can go out to eat and to a movie. Here's some money."

Gracie told me that my uncle, looking bewildered, shook his head and refused to take it. They immediately left the house, returning later that night only after all the cars for the party had departed. They left for good early the next morning, never to visit again.

Horrified, Gracie wanted to confront Mom about how rude she had been to her own brother. Like me, Gracie struggled with an inner conflict of wanting to confront Mom versus wanting to keep things as peaceful as possible during a spell. The peace option always won. We knew from experience Mom would insist that what she said, or what she did made perfect sense. Unfortunately, it often made sense only to her. Seeing her proper manners replaced by abrupt, inconsiderate or rude actions during a spell baffled both Gracie and me. We wondered why she sometimes acted like this. What was wrong with her?

A few days later, Gracie and I were eating breakfast when Mom announced in an excited voice, "Girls, we are going to have a backyard supper for about twenty people. Next Saturday night." Gracie and I rolled our eyes at each other.

Mom's Spells

Other people thought Mom's parties were heaps of fun as her creativity engaged her guests in all types of activities, like pinning the name of a famous person on each person's back. They had to guess who it was by asking the other guests a series of questions.

Gracie and I now knew Mom's spell was turning super-hyper and what that meant. The yard, terraces, garage, windows and entire house must be cleaned, swept, dusted, straightened, raked or washed before the party. Tables and chairs had to be picked up from various friends. Silverware polished. Tablecloths and napkins starched and ironed. The menu decided, changed, bought and prepped.

Our one-day-a-week housekeeper worked an extra day, but most of the preparation fell to Gracie and me. Dad disappeared in the direction of the hospital or the golf course. That week, we spent every waking moment before and after school fetching or cleaning. I cancelled my plan to go to the movies with my girlfriends Friday night.

Invitations were issued and guests added to the list. As the day of the party approached, the phone rang incessantly. Mom announced, "We need another table. Diane, call and see if Jessie has another one. And four folding chairs. Gracie, go get them. If not, call Annie and see if she has extras."

"No, no, no. That's all wrong. Put the tables over there. And clean the hurricane lamp chimneys again. You left smudges all over them. No, no. Don't put the napkins on the plates. Do it this way. Don't do it that way. Do it all over," she said in reference to everything we did.

Mom's actions became even more frantic. She started talking to herself. Strange things occurred.

I was re-cleaning the lamp chimneys at the kitchen counter when Mom opened the refrigerator door. "What are these scissors doing in the refrigerator?" she asked, tiny eyebrows raised.

"You must have put them there Mom," I replied. "Were you planning on making cold cuts?"

She didn't laugh.

THE DAY OF THE PARTY was predictable. We were all exhausted and of course something always went wrong. Any little glitch became a major catastrophe.

"NO, OH NO." I heard Mom wail from the kitchen. I ran in and saw the reason why. The water in the pot of green beans had boiled over, flooding the stove top with hot water. Mom started moving the other pots off the stove onto the yellow tiled counter top, muttering, "OhdearOhdearOhdear." I turned off all the heating elements of the electric stove and Mom started trying to mop up the water with several cloth dishrags but they were too hot to pick up.

"Here," I said, handing her some tongs, "use these to put them in the sink. I'll run cold water over them before I squeeze them out."

Working as a team, we managed to clear up the stove mess, but then the floor needed to be mopped and all the food put back on to cook. It took about fifteen minutes, making all the food prep behind schedule.

Mom's tension escalated as she proceeded in a dither, becoming more and more irrational as the party time approached. Just before the guests arrived, Mom flung herself on her bed, still in her undies, and burst into tears. "It is all ruined, my party's ruined."

The doorbell rang. Dad went to greet the guests.

Twenty minutes later Mom made a grand entrance to her own party, looking lovely and excited. And party she did. Two hours later while Gracie and I were finishing the dishes we could hear her laughing, and talking rapidly in her party voice.

The next day we started taking everything back, dreading the next party announcement. It came three days later. "Girls, I'm going to have a bridge party next Tuesday afternoon. Won't that be fun? About three tables. And let's think, what can I serve? Lunch? Or maybe just dessert. Yes. Something special. Something chocolate. I'll serve Annie's yummy chocolate pecan pie recipe. With ice cream on top of each piece. And a cherry.

"Gracie, did you return Jessie's card table and chairs yet? If you did, call her and go get them again."

Another week into this spell, our fun-loving Party Mom started turning into a tense demanding person no one could please. She yelled more, criticized more and demanded instant responses to her commands. Tension vibrated through the house. While I no longer feared being whipped, I flinched under her frequent caustic critiques.

"Why didn't you get straight A's? You should be getting A's like I used to.

"Sweep the porch again. Can't you do anything right? Look over there. You left some sand under that chair leg.

"Diane, you're slumping. Stand up straight. Straighter.

"You're not going to the movie until you finish that pile of ironing. And do a better job on the napkins. You left too many wrinkles last week."

The tension ratcheted up day by day. Frown lines stayed between Mom's flashing, angry eyes. Her criticisms escalated into loud tirades. Her frantic, angry words and body signals warned me to vanish. I did.

It never occurred to either Gracie or me to refuse to help her or not do what she dictated. Mom had us well trained—we always obeyed silently. Even though none of the jobs she ever had me do were onerous, I felt my resentments grow. I didn't have any problem doing what she asked me to do—just doing them to her expectations.

Didn't Mom realize she would never have a perfect party or a perfect daughter? One syllable of praise for even one thing I did to help her would have gone a long way in making me happier to do any of them. I kept longing for any word of approval. I don't recall any. Ever. Where were the "thank yous" she trained me to say to others? Didn't I count as a person who should sometimes be thanked? Evidently not. She seemed to always be stuck in one mode of communication to me—what I did wrong.

Despite my feeling of despair of being incapable and incompetent in Mom's eyes, down deep in my core, a tiny spark of confidence still flickered. I had to believe that she was wrong. I had to believe that one day I would do something wonderful, something special and she would say something nice to me.

ONE AFTERNOON I STARTED WORKING in the utility room on a relief map of the United States for my geography class. It took longer than I expected. In the middle of molding the Rocky Mountains with globs of wet plaster mixed with sawdust, I heard Mom call, "Diane, it's time to set the table."

"I'm finishing my map." I yelled back.

"Dinner's almost ready. YOU COME HERE RIGHT NOW AND GET THAT TABLE SET."

The puny mountain range needed to be wider and longer. I grabbed the bucket and plopped more plaster goop on Wyoming, trying to build the Rockies up fast, my hands all gooey and sticky. When I didn't show up immediately I heard her frequent threat, "WAIT TILL YOUR FATHER COMES HOME."

I left the half-formed mountain range, knowing that my project wouldn't get a good grade and hurried to scrub my hands and the bucket in the laundry sink before appearing in the breakfast room.

Jaw clenched, I grabbed the plates out of the cabinet, ready to slam them on the table. Then I stopped. To gain control of my anger I stared at the one wallpaper seam in the breakfast room where the paperhanger had misaligned the small colorful flowers. Blowing out a huff, I slowly counted the mismatched flowers until my anger abated. I set the table, dreading the next ten minutes.

The four of us sat down to eat, covered our laps with the cloth napkins I had carefully ironed, and bowed our heads for the blessing.

Then IT started.

"Edward, I don't know what I am going to do about Diane . . ."

I focused on Critical Mom's crimson lips as all my transgressions for the day spewed out of them, one appalling description after another. Each event had a basis of truth, but hearing Mom's rendition of my shortcomings, one would think I was deliberately disobeying her.

Dad listened, frowned, then without a comment, reached over and thumped me hard on my temple. Waves of sharp pain shot through my head.

I sat there. Stunned. Shocked. Tears flooded my eyes. My head pounded. Throbbed.

I didn't try to make Mom mad, especially during the irritable parts of a spell. It was just impossible to please her. And worst of all now Dad thought I misbehaved on purpose.

Prosecutor Mom's accounting of my transgressions to Judge Daddy occurred night after night for the next ten days. No defense was allowed. I sat there mute, head bowed, awaiting my punishment, feeling unjustly accused and powerless to escape this nightly ordeal.

Some nights Dad just sighed and shook his head, evidently very disappointed with me. Thump or no thump, my heart broke.

Gracie never received this treatment as she tried harder and succeeded more often in living up to Mom's impossible demands. But I noticed that while Mom seldom criticized Gracie, she didn't compliment or thank her either.

If Perfect Gracie couldn't please Mom, what hope did I have? Why try? I would always fail in her eyes.

I started to wonder if I was just one child too many. Or one girl too many. I put five and five together, recalling when I was five and Mom told us she had been praying for five years to have a son. She had hoped I would be a boy. I had been failing to meet Mom's expectations ever since my first cry.

Feeling totally incapable of ever living up to Mom's expectations, I brooded. Resentment grew. The seeds of rebellion sprouted roots.

Finally, Dad put a stop to the nightly accusations during dinner, announcing to us all, "Dinnertime is not the place for correcting Diane." Corrections didn't come later either. I think he finally figured out my sins were worse in Mom's mixed-up head than in reality. He seemed to understand I took the brunt of Mom's ire during her spells and occasionally gave me a little hug when he left for the day, or arrived home. My heart soared each time. Daddy did care about me even if Mom didn't.

WHILE THE BEGINNINGS OF MOM'S spells were typically heralded by obvious changes in her behavior, the endings were less obvious. As that school year ended I felt less tense and realized that Mom seemed less angry, less agitated. Her irritated rebukes, tirades and marathon talking sprees gradually waned. Gracie and I hoped months and months would pass before the inevitable happened and she started winding up again.

I wondered each time we survived another spell: Why? Why does she have them?

THANKFULLY THIS SPELL ENDED BY the time the summer of 1952 started and we discovered I had a serious medical problem.

6

Mom's Help

L OOKING IN THE FULL-LENGTH MIRROR on Mom's bathroom door, I studied my figure in my new white swimsuit. I turned to view all my angles, checking to see if it showed the curves that had started developing before my twelfth birthday. But the curve I noticed turned out to be a surprise. One of my protruding hip bones looked obviously higher than the other one.

"Mom, I'm crooked," I said.

"Stand up straight."

"I am standing up straight. I'm crooked. Look. LOOK AT ME." She finally glanced up from her desk and stared.

"Why Diane, you are crooked."

Dad viewed many x-rays of my spine taken from all angles. It had started to curve into a distinct S shape. Trips to orthopedic specialists in Dallas resulted in more x-rays. The diagnosis was scoliosis, a curvature of the spine that if not corrected could threaten major organs. I would develop an obvious deformity like a lopsided humped back.

Deformed. A lump formed in my throat and stuck there.

MOM AND I SAT IN chairs before the surgeon's desk in his office in Dallas. After a phone conference, Dad had stayed home to work instead of attending this follow-up visit for some additional tests. As the doctor started to explain about the required surgery, Mom motioned for me to leave. I started to get up.

"No," the surgeon said, "I want her to hear what is to be done. She needs to know what is going to happen to her."

I sat back down, fearful, a pounding in my ears making his voice seem far away. I didn't understand all of the medical terms or details, but I did grasp

Mom's Help 63

I had to have back surgery, miss a half-year of school, and be in a body cast for nine months. The surgery would be done in September.

As the best specialist to do this type of surgery was in Dallas, this presented a problem. I could not be left alone in the hospital for the weeks required to do all the preparation, surgery and recovery. Dad could not leave his practice that long. Thus, Mom accompanied me, even though she was scared to stay in a hotel by herself at night.

After checking into the hospital, I discovered it would be two weeks before the surgery. During the wait, I started to look like a white wrapped mummy. They encased me in a total body cast that wrapped around the back of my head, under my chin and around my whole torso and down my left leg to the knee. At least it was sleeveless. After it dried, large diamond-shaped sections were cut out of each side of the cast. Turnbuckles were installed and adjusted to create a curve in the cast. Changes occurred daily until x-rays confirmed the major curve in my spine was now immobilized in the straightest line possible.

Mom and I settled into a routine. She stayed in the little hotel across the street and came over early to help me eat breakfast each morning. Eating presented a challenge as I could only lie flat on my back or my right side, impeding my arm. I tried to feed myself, but made a mess. Soup and English peas presented an impossible challenge. There was just no way I could keep from tilting the spoon sideways.

The endless hours stretched into marathon long, boring days. Television was not available in hospital rooms yet. To relieve the tedium, Mom rigged a hand mirror to the trapeze bar over my orthopedic bed so I could at least see out the window. I spent hours watching a parking lot being paved across the street—very exciting. At least I could lose myself in books, taking a break every fifteen minutes as my arms tired from holding them up. After my dinner at 5:00, Mom would leave to eat an early dinner so that she could lock herself in her hotel room before dark. Staying by my bedside all day and by herself at night, in a hotel, in a strange city, must have been very difficult for her, a fact I didn't appreciate at the time.

Midmorning, the day before my surgery, a male orderly entered my hospital room announcing he was there to shave me.

"Shave me? What for?" I asked, increasingly apprehensive about the imminent surgery.

"We shave the surgical area because hair can have bacteria on it that can cause an infection and we want to avoid that." I looked at Mom, then nodded assent as best I could in my plaster helmet.

"Let me help you turn over," he said, reaching out, helping me maneuver onto my stomach with my head hanging off the bed so I could breathe.

The orderly untaped the plaster door that had been cut in the back of my cast for the surgery. Free from the heat of the Plaster of Paris, my back felt a delightful draft of fresh air. I heard water swishing in a pan as he explained, "I am going to soap your back now." Ohhhh, the wet soapy cloth felt incredible on my hot, dry, itchy skin. I wanted it to last longer. "Hold still." A gentle touch of something. It must be the razor. I kept still, unable to wiggle my back if I wanted to. A dry rough towel wiped my back as he said, "All done," and taped my cast back together. Mom had not said a word–very unusual.

"I need you to turn back over now so I can shave your leg."

I heard Mom gasp.

"Shave my leg? Why?" I asked, rolling onto my side, grabbing the trapeze bar and flipping onto my back. "I'm not having an operation on my leg." He consulted the chart and confirmed that my right leg was to be shaved along my calf.

"Mom, tell him it is just my back, not my leg," I whimpered, frightened over this unexpected news. I saw her motioning to the orderly, shaking her head.

"MOM!" She wouldn't look at me. A wave of panic hit me. Instantly I wanted out of that cast, out of that bed, out of that hospital. She finally looked at me and confirmed what she had decided not to tell me.

In a subdued voice she admitted, "They need to place chips of bone from your leg between your vertebras for the fusion. Your Dad offered to have them use his bone, but they said it was best to use your own. They are going to have to take some bone chips from your leg."

I lay there stunned, mute, my heart thudding against my cast. Why didn't she tell me? Did she expect me to wake up and not notice that my leg was cut open? What other secrets would I wake up and discover?

Staring at Mom, I felt my tummy churn. Anger swept down my entire body. Then Fear. Cold Fear.

Dad arrived that evening, his calm demeanor comforting. The next morning he was permitted to be with me during the operation. The last thing I saw before the lights went out was my dad, by my side, holding my hand.

Finally it was over and I discovered what Mom had tried to keep from me. Twenty-five, horrible, ugly stitches closed the incision that went from my knee to my ankle down my painfully swollen right leg. Moving it even an inch elicited a piercing scream from me. My leg was going to have a huge ugly scar. Forever.

A week later, back home via ambulance, I settled into a hospital ortho-pedic bed in our den, among the fifteen houseplants I used to water weekly. My new routine included school work so I wouldn't fall behind my peers. Teachers visited weekly with lesson plans. Since writing while on my back was impossible and turning on my right side resulted in illegible scribbles, Mom became my scribe. She seemed to enjoy being my tutor. I soon noticed any wrong answer I gave resulted in her saying, "Think again." We received very good grades.

Gracie helped by taking over the feed-Diane routine and even slept every night on a roll-away bed in the den. I got scared in there by myself. Howling Texas winds, spooky wavy shadows and too many doorways made me feel vulnerable, trapped in that cast, in case of fire or burglars. I felt safer with Gracie nearby.

Totally bedridden, I listened daily to my chief source of entertainment—a radio. It was 1952, a presidential election year. After listening to hours of political speeches and commentators, I decided I liked Ike—the general who commanded the invasion that defeated Hitler. I also decided I would marry someone who would become President of the United States. I would become the First Lady. It didn't occur to me in that era that I could be the President. Of course my daydream didn't happen, but that election sparked a lasting interest in national politics.

The most challenging times during my convalescence included bedpan, bath and hair washing times. Never once did I hear Nurse Mom complain as she took care of my every bodily need. Nor did she complain about giving up her social life, clubs, church or gardening during those bed-ridden months as the bone transplants between my six vertebrae started to solidify into one continuous inflexible bone.

As an almost teen, I assumed that my family would help me through this ordeal; that they would be there when I needed anything. I don't recall thinking much about what they gave up, or my ever thanking them. It has only been in retrospect that I fully appreciate how they all adjusted their lives to take care of me and how their actions showed they cared, including Mom.

We were lucky she didn't have a spell during these months.

Three months later we went back to Dallas for a cast change. This cast was strapless and only encased my torso. I could walk, but I had to learn how again. Wow, the first time I tried to stand on my feet it felt like my heel bones were poking right through the tender skin on my feet. Trying to take steps, I couldn't tolerate putting my weight on one foot for long, so I hopped from one foot to the other like Wile E. Coyote after the Road Runner gives him a hot foot.

NONE OF MY PRETTY CLOTHES fit over my cast. Mom went shopping for loose clothes and larger panties plus other items she considered essential.

She reached into the shopping bag and pulled out a thickly padded white bra.

"Oh no. I'm not going to wear falsies."

"Yes, you are. You want to look nice, normal. And falsies will help you do that." she replied, giving me the padded bra. It would have to be worn over my torso-encompassing cast. I hated it.

As my thick, full-torso cast made my figure look like a stuffed barrel, my new wardrobe consisted of huge wrap-around dresses. A wide elastic belt held them closed. Real cute. It was mortifying enough going to junior high wearing a cast and those stupid-looking old lady clothes without putting false breasts on. Mom insisted. Off I went, the two pointy pads sticking out of my plastered chest area. They often slid up toward my collarbones. Of course I couldn't feel that happening through my cast. Giggles from my friends let me know when I needed an adjustment.

Ah, the agony of looking different when you are almost a teenager. Bumping and clunking into things for the next six months, I watched with envy as my friends' bodies changed shapes, with soft curves—in all the right places.

The escape from my plaster cocoon wasn't like a butterfly suddenly emerging in stunning beauty. My bosom, blossoming prior to the cast, had been compressed for nine months and no longer existed. Straightening my spine and a growth spurt had added four inches to my height. Weighing only one hundred pounds at five feet eight inches, I looked anorexic, the antitheses of Marilyn Monroe and voluptuous curves that were the current vogue.

Without the heavy protective cast I felt physically vulnerable, but mentally liberated. After ten months I was at last free of hospitals, X-rays, doctors and Mom's constant scrutiny. Free. Finally free of the stigma of looking different, and of being crooked. My life as a teenager could now begin. But not without a critical comment from Mom.

"Diane, go put your falsies on. You look absolutely flat-chested."

"But Mom, I have them on."

7

Teen Angst: Confrontation # 1

AS A PRETEEN FULL OF romantic ideas, I thought my parents were horribly mismatched. Dad was quiet, calm and retiring; Mom lively, social, unpredictable. He could be counted on in a crisis; she went into a dither.

How did my two very different parents ever get married? Mom told me about the series of events that created their chance meeting. She said, "I planned to become a schoolteacher after going to the junior college in my hometown. But when I applied for a teaching job, the school director took me out in the country to an isolated one-room school house. I was expected to live in the attached teacher's quarters. I took one look at the dark, foreboding forest surrounding it and told him, I can't stay here by myself. Take me back.

"After that, with financial help from my uncle, I moved to Houston to attend the Jeff Davis Hospital School of Nursing. My parents' didn't want me to go, but I knew I needed to get good skills to get a good job.

"It wasn't long before I got attention from the faculty. I wowed them with papers using footnoted references. In my final paper I told them everything currently wrong with nurses' training and what they should do about it. We were treated as little more than maids in the 1930s. We were required to sweep and mop the floors, made the beds, wash the linens and the windows plus bathe, bed-pan and medicate the patients. It was exhausting work."

Immediately after she graduated, the Administrator asked Dixie to become the Assistant Supervisor of Nurses at that huge charity hospital. "I decided to take the position only after I completed some graduate work at The Mayo Hospital in Minnesota. I knew that my classmates wouldn't want me to supervise them unless I had further training. I returned a year later and took that post."

One day at noon, just as she started to shut the door to her office, the phone rang. She stopped, hesitated, then turned back from the doorway and answered the phone.

"We need you at the second floor nurses' station. There is a question about the meds for one of our patients."

After solving the problem, Dixie checked her watch. She had missed half her lunch period. Hurrying, she headed to the stairwell and started downstairs. Halfway down, she spied a new blonde intern in his spiffy white doctor's coat coming up the stairs. He spotted her about the same time. Steps slowed. Eyes locked. Pheromones flared, igniting an instant reaction in both of them.

He grinned at the slim nurse with the dark hair. She was pretty. Very pretty. She grinned back.

He said, "I'm lost in this huge hospital. How about showing me around?" The sparkling diamond on her left hand didn't deter him for even one second—nor did it hinder her response.

"I get off at 4:00. Is that soon enough?"

EDWARD WAS COMPLETING HIS INTERNSHIP after working his way through medical school during the depression. He had grown up in East Texas, on a poor dairy farm that had a herd of only six cows. His hard-working mother encouraged him often, saying, "Son, get an education so you don't have to live like this."

Not long after that chance meeting, and the evening spent getting acquainted that followed, Edward started walking into Dixie's office daily to snap off the live blossom she had put in a bud vase on her desk. Placing it in his buttonhole, he would flash her a flirtatious grin and exit without saying a word.

Within a week of their meeting Mom returned the engagement ring to her fiancé in Minnesota. Only five months after their initial stairway encounter, my parents married.

After Edward's graduation, the newlyweds loaded their belongings—a floor radio, two table lamps, linens and wedding crystal into Mom's navy coupe and moved to dry, windblown North Creek, Texas. There Dad went into practice with a doctor who owned a small five bed hospital. My sister arrived the next year. I followed two-and-a-half years later.

If Dixie had not been scared to stay by herself in that schoolhouse at night—or gone to lunch on time that day, Gracie and I might not exist.

I WONDERED: DID MOM HAVE spells even then? Did my parents meet in the lull between spells during those five months of courtship? Or did they meet during her playful weeks at the beginning of a spell when her inhibitions evaporated? When did Dad first meet Hyper Mom? After the wedding? After my birth?

Years later I understood their relationship better. Edward brought stability to Dixie's life; she brought excitement to his. As true opposites, they enhanced each other's lives. He was the centerboard, she the sail, unfortunately sometimes propelled by volatile winds.

ALTHOUGH NEITHER GRACIE NOR I ever heard our parents argue or witnessed a disagreement between them, their relationship wasn't without problems. When we were preteens, they had a crisis that threatened their marriage. It probably occurred during one of Mom's spells. Gracie picked up on the tension between them.

After Dad left abruptly on an unplanned trip and Mom's eyes looked red and swollen, Gracie became a sleuth. She retrieved a letter Mom had drafted and thrown in the wastebasket. Of course we read it. Covered with scratched out words, her attempt to apologize didn't reveal what had happened, but it may have been the event Mom told me about later to warn me about the evils of alcohol.

She said, "We both used to drink cocktails, especially at parties. During a party at a friend's house, I had a bit too much to drink. I headed to the master bedroom to retrieve my lipstick from my purse on the bed, and to use the bathroom. A man who had been flirting with me, followed me, pulled me into the bathroom, closed the door and made a pass at me. Laughing, I pushed him away and opened the door. There stood your father, stone-faced. We left immediately. I never took one sip of alcohol from that moment forth.

Teen Angst: Confrontation # 1

"The moral to this," she admonished me, "is that you should never drink. Even a little bit of alcohol can create situations where you do things you would not consider doing sober. In an instant you can destroy something precious."

I suspected that Mom's flirty actions at that party probably gave that man the idea she would welcome his pass. Later I learned that liquor, mixed with spells like mom's, creates a volatile cocktail that triggers many regrettable, impulsive actions harmful to relationships and families.

MY TEEN YEARS WERE NOT easy ones in our family. As Mom was thirty at the time of my birth, by the time my hormones started flowing in one direction, her hormones started flowing in reverse. Hot flashes kept interrupting her sleep. She became agitated and demanding. Tensions spiraled. Spells happened. When she became hyper, the chaotic hormone mix in our home became even more explosive. Even Diane-the-Vanishing couldn't escape every negative comment.

"Your curfew is 10:00 o'clock. I don't care if the movie doesn't end until 10:15. You leave in time to be in this house by 10:00. NOT A MINUTE LATER."

"Your hair, your hair. Why can't you do something with it?"

"That isn't enough salad for eight people. Put some more of everything in it. Can't you do anything right?"

"You girls. You girls. I don't know what I am going to do with you."

"You are not going anywhere in that get-up. Go put on that yellow dress I bought you last week."

Why, I wondered, does Mom always have to be so critical? Her daily score: negative comments toward me—seven; positive comments or any sign of affection—zero.

I felt like Cinderella, dressed in clothes I didn't want to wear and always having to finish some task before I could go have fun. Resentment built.

"WHAT WILL PEOPLE SAY?" WE heard Mom's recurring mantra over and over, except during her spells. Many times, observing that her headstrong demands had obviously upset someone, I thought: you don't have a clue what people are really saying about you. If you paid any attention you would know they think you are demanding and bossy, always insisting that people do things your way. You're totally unaware that you say things that upset them or hurt their feelings. People roll their eyes and shake their heads behind your back. Why, why, why do you act this way?

When I couldn't get up the gumption to confront Mom with the impact of her actions on others—or me—I railed at myself. Berated myself. I continued to spend futile hours having imaginary confrontations with her, like the time I came close to pleading with her to shut up after listening to her incessant jabbering, but once again, I chose to shut myself up.

Being a wimp took a lot of energy. I often felt emotionally exhausted trying to live up to Mom's demands, her insistence that Gracie and I have perfect manners, perfect hair, perfect grades.

The harder I tried to be perfect in Mom's eyes, the more each of her criticisms irritated me. So why even try? Sensing that pleasing Mom was never going to happen, I started developing a "who cares" attitude and withdrew even more, eating meals in silence—my own, not hers. I did my tasks, went to my room and shut the door rather than spend evenings near her watching our first television set. At least sharing a room with Gracie provided a quiet, peaceful place of safety to study or read. We sisters also shared a goal—to survive in silence and compliance—until we could get away from her.

I never complained to my friends about how difficult living with Mom had become, and rarely invited them over for fear Mom would embarrass me. One told me recently, "We became nervous at your house. We all knew we had to be on our best behavior around your mother."

Gracie, the only other person who knew what being Dixie's child was like, would soon escape to college. I still occasionally fantasized that a real Prince Charming would appear and rescue me. I ached with emotional needs. What I wanted, more than anything, was for someone to hold me, to make me feel loved. Wanted. Cherished.

DAD HAD NOT BEEN AROUND much during the early years of my life. While a pleasant Dad, not harsh or critical like Mom, he had not related easily to young children. Gracie and I still rarely saw him except during breakfast or dinner. Now that we were teens, he tried to interest us in his passion—golf.

He played golf on the three afternoons the clinic closed: Wednesday, Saturday and Sunday. After Gracie and I finished a series of golf lessons on the rocky, almost bare dirt public golf course, we headed out to the Country

Teen Angst: Confrontation # 1   73

Club to play a round of nine holes with Dad and Mom, also a novice player. At least this club had grass on the fairways.

On the first tee, Gracie hit her ball fairly well. It even went up in the air. Mine, well it made headway along the ground. Mom's? She managed to whiff her ball the first try, but then swinging as hard as she could she hit it down the fairway. Dad's ball went high and long, almost out of sight.

On the next series of shots Mom swung at her ball. Missed. Realigned. Swung harder. Missed again. Mustering up all her strength she swung so hard her feet flew out from under her. Up in the air she went, landing on her backside with her feet in the air. What a sight. Even she burst into giggles. Gracie and I laughed so hard we cried. What a rare and special moment: the four Dwellers sharing a family laugh.

The golf bug either bites or it doesn't. While neither Gracie nor I felt that bite, we did enjoy family-night putting contests and even scored fairly well. Thus, we did share some time with Dad—but does a daughter ever think it's enough?

BY MY SOPHOMORE YEAR IN high school I became determined to get out from under Mom's control over what I wore. Jeans, or lack thereof, became the catalyst for my first, long-planned, long-awaited confrontation. Everybody wore jeans on Fridays, the only day girls were allowed to wear pants to school in the mid-1950s. Mom didn't permit us to wear jeans on any day.

"Please, please let me wear jeans on Fridays," I begged her over and over.

"No. You girls are not boys and you are going to dress like ladies and wear a proper skirt or dress."

I planned my revolt carefully. I saved up birthday money and bought a pair of boy's jeans as female proportioned jeans would not be available for years. After sneaking them into the house, I put them on, sat in a tub of *very* hot water, sneaked out of the house with the squishy, soggy jeans on. I wore them until they had dried—thus shrinking and stretching them to fit my female shape—and ensuring they could not be returned.

The next Friday morning, heart pounding, I entered the kitchen, hoping Mom would not notice my jeans. She looked up from the stove and instantly demanded, "What are you wearing? WHAT DO YOU HAVE ON?"

"Jeans," I said with a toss of my head.

"YOU ARE NOT WEARING THOSE JEANS TO SCHOOL." In a flash, Mom's face contorted into Scary Mom's.

"Yes, I am." I stared at her, jaw clenched, adrenaline and alarm both surging through every cell in my body. "Everybody in Texas wears jeans except you."

"You are not going to school in those jeans. TAKE THEM OFF RIGHT NOW."

We stood there glaring at each other. I started to waver, then a huge surge of built-up defiance flooded my body. "NO. I WON'T. AND YOU CAN'T MAKE ME."

I saw a blur, then felt the sting of her hand on my cheek as my head snapped back. I crashed backwards into the kitchen counter. Pain shot up my fused spine. Lurching up, I glared at her and shrieked, "I HATE YOU. HATE YOU. HATE YOU."

Running past the maid, I fled down the hall into my bedroom, slamming the door shut. Sinking to the floor beside my bed, seething and shocked at her slap, I felt my stinging cheek. I sat there rocking back and forth, hugging my knees, hugging my hate, fighting off an overwhelming urge to crawl under my bed and count the slats.

Gracie, sitting on her bed, had heard the confrontation. She kept quiet, her eyes big.

Mom entered shortly without knocking.

"Do you have anything to say to me?" she asked, her tone hard and ugly.

I didn't answer. I truly did hate her. Hated my life with her. I wanted out of her life. OUT. NOW.

Her next comment made me even madder. "Aren't you sorry you said that in front of the maid?" Obviously what the maid thought ranked higher than me or my feelings. Of her slapping me.

When I didn't respond, she left our room. I left for school with Gracie, wearing my new jeans, defying Mom totally. She saw me. Looked hurt. Totally disapproving. I didn't care. I left, feeling the sting of that slap in my heart.

Every Friday thereafter, I tugged on those jeans with a sense of martyrdom and defiantly made sure Mom saw that I had them on. She never said another word about them, but every Friday the frown on her face and her tight lips conveyed that I was a major disappointment, a terrible daughter.

Had Mom ever politely said, "Please don't wear those jeans to school," I probably would have begrudgingly changed clothes.

Even though I had at last broken her dictatorship over what I had to wear, my victory felt hollow. While winning my first overt battle with Mom, I found myself capitulating on other issues after that slap.

It would be three decades before I directly confronted her again—in a very strange and different way.

When I became furious with Mom during my teen years, I often disappeared, not under my bed, but to an outcropping of sandstone boulders around the hill behind our house. Standing on the largest bolder, I would vent my rage at the cloudless sky. Punching the air with clenched fists, I filled the air with my fury.

"Why, why, why can't I go?"

"Stop criticizing me."

"Why is everything I do wrong? I try so hard to do things the way you want them."

Looking down the hill and across the street, I often spied the three shaggy buffalo that lived in the fenced acreage. They didn't even turn their heads at my shouts. The only response to my cries came from the metal windmill that suppled them with water. It echoed my groans as it rotated in the breeze.

Finally calm, emotionally drained, breathing deeper, I would feel the tension slowly seeping from my body. As the gentle breeze dried the tears on my cheeks, each deep breath, full of fragrance from the cedar and sage bushes, helped me cope with yet another bad-Mom-moment.

Sinking down on my favorite stone seat, I found it hard to stay angry and upset while surrounded by Mother Nature's peace and quiet. I often picked up one of the long nails cached nearby and once more carved my initials deeper into the sandstone. I dared to dream of the freedom I would have once I left home and Mom far behind. When I finally did escape at age seventeen, deep grooves spelled out my initials plus several shallow initials of the boys I had once hoped would love me.

Even today, when upset, it only takes nanoseconds for me to mentally retreat to the tranquility of my sandstone sanctuary, my mental refuge on this turbulent globe spinning through space.

Since the end of my piano failure years before, I had periodically begged to take art lessons. Art was not offered in our public schools, but finally, after I started high school, Mom relented and agreed to private lessons. While my local teacher lacked any major talent, she did show me how mixing two colors could make countless more hues. Take a blob of yellow, add a tiny bit of red and you get a pale orange. Yellow plus a little violet resulted in the murky color of Texas dirt. I could make countless new colors. What joy. The hours with a paint brush in my hand flew by even when Mom decided what I had to paint: a poem about roses, some picture-presents for relatives, even a design on a tie for an uncle. Each finished picture resulted in a critique or no comment at all. She would sometimes stare at my painting and then hand it back to me with no expression.

I thought about painting her a picture of roses surrounding the words 'An ounce of praise goes further than a pound of criticism.' The word criticism would be surrounded with sharp-thorned cactus. But I didn't.

Creating new colors, tints and shades with my paints every week, I started to imagine what colors I would paint people. I'd paint Mom in explosive colors, all hot red with fiery yellow streaks. Dad would be a cool blue; Gracie, coral with glowing sunrise golds. Me? I'd paint my outside a dull gray but underneath it would be my rebellious streak—flashes of vibrant hot pink with an occasional white lightning stroke.

I had fun when I let my true colors show. Secret mutiny against Mom's strict code of conduct became my way of rebelling against her. The thrill of doing what I knew she would disapprove of tempted me more than once—like when my table-mates in the cooking class at school were in charge of making the eggnog, minus the nog, for the teacher's Christmas party. Having been taught to carefully follow recipes by our teacher, I thought we should add the nog. So, I sneaked out a bottle of booze given to Dad by a patient. Giggling, three conspirators kept a lookout as the liquor went glug, glug, glug into the creamy punch.

The whole faculty raved, "This eggnog is the best ever." Even the timid librarian came back for seconds.

When school resumed in January, the home economics teacher, staring hard at me, remarked she had learned that someone had spiked the eggnog.

Teen Angst: Confrontation # 1

Somebody snitched, but punishment was averted. Thank goodness all the evidence had been consumed—with gusto.

Since Mom's beauty garnered attention and compliments for her, it obviously upset her that her daughters were not beauties. We tried over and over to please her with our appearances, only to hear daily comments like these:

"Take that sweater off. It looks awful with that skirt."

"Pull your top down even. You look sloppy."

"Why are you wearing those shoes? Your white sandals will look better. Go change."

"Go fix your hair."

"Put on some lipstick. You look dead without it."

Though sisters with similar facial features, Gracie and I were very different. Younger by two-and-a-half years, I ended up two inches taller. Our differences didn't stop with our auburn and light brown hair colors; we also had different temperaments. Gracie became a cheerful extrovert, an overachiever, excellent student and compliant daughter. I became introverted, watchful and wary, inwardly rebellious.

Tact was not Mom's long suit, especially during a spell when she became brutally honest. Although she admonished us not to say anything if we could not say something nice, that advice did not apply to her. She was just stating the truth.

Gracie and I arrived home from school one day and headed to the kitchen for a snack. Mom looked up from her chair in the breakfast room, watched us a few minutes, then announced, "I saw Mildred's two daughters today. They are both so beautiful." She stared at us. Then shook her head. We got that message.

Mom didn't get this message: She was in the middle of the cranky part of a spell that had lasted several weeks when my sister, now a senior in high school, came home flushed and excited with some news. Heading immediately into the kitchen she jubilantly announced, "Mom, I've been voted one of the five school beauty finalists this year."

Mom turned from the sink and stared at Gracie for a long moment. "Well," she said, "they must have counted the votes wrong." Without another word, she turned back to the sink.

Gracie looked like Mom had slapped her.

I gasped. How could she be so cruel?

I DIDN'T BOTHER TO TELL Mom when I also received the same honor in my senior year. She found out when she saw my picture in the Sunday paper.

"Why didn't you tell me?" she asked.

I shrugged my shoulders, hoping for a smile of approval but expecting a comment about how they miscounted the votes. She shook her head, looking confused about how this mistake had been made again.

I thought, if I were selected Miss Texas and then Miss America and then Miss Universe, I bet Mom would still find a way to make me feel plain and ugly.

Later Mom assured Gracie that even plain girls could get a nice husband.

How about a nice mother?

WHILE MY FEELINGS OF FAILURE and inadequacy continued at home, at school it became a different story. Each good grade gave me confidence that I could do something right. And when my peers selected me for several honors during my high school years, I thought with surprise, people do like me, even if Mom doesn't. With each social and scholastic achievement, my fragile self-esteem started to change into confidence—away from Mom.

I became successful in positions of leadership at both school and church where one of the unexpected benefits turned out to be the Sunday evening Bible Study Class. We were required to speak assigned parts in front of the group every Sunday night. Over time, my shaky knees and quivery voice morphed into presenting my parts with confidence and joy. I didn't know then how important this training would be in my future.

DATING UNDER DIXIE'S SHARP EYES presented challenges. She kept repeating her rules: "Do not ever, ever call a boy, and never, never beat a boy at any game. Stay out of back seats and off of their laps. If they drink any liquor, you are to call us to come and get you."

Teen Angst: Confrontation # 1

Dating in the Fifties consisted of innocent fun. We teens had great times, mainly going to the one movie house in town or the drive-in, hanging out at the Dairy Queen or playing Putt-Putt.

One night after prepping for my date to a movie with Jerry, I took a last look in the mirror on the closet door, checking out my appearance in my favorite Lanz dress with the tiny blue flowers. Trying to fluff up my hair a little more, I saw car lights flash outside. Peeking out the bedroom window, I grinned as I saw Jerry strolling up the sidewalk looking great in snug jeans and a crisp short-sleeved shirt with the sleeves rolled-up. Hurrying through the den and living room, I reached the front door about the time he rang the doorbell. I let him in, feeling my pulse quicken at the sight of his curly brown hair and hazel eyes. He grinned.

"Good evening Jerry," Mom called from the adjacent jungle-den.

Holding hands, we went and stood before her to get our instructions.

"Nice to see you, Jerry. You know you are to have Diane home no later than ten o'clock?"

"Yes Ma'am."

"Not a minute later."

"Yes Ma'am." he responded, bobbing his head. He turned and nodded at Dad too, "Evening sir."

We exited as quickly as possible.

We saw a scary movie about nuclear war with Russia. The scenes seemed frightening and real. The Cold War with Russia that could turn hot was a reality in the late Fifties. The schools held duck-and-cover drills where we crouched down in the hallways and put our hands over our heads to minimize the impact of atomic bomb fallout.

As Jerry and I sat in the darkened theater, dramatic music swelled. Our planes, loaded with nuclear weapons were approaching Moscow to start a nuclear holocaust when I glanced at the clock on the wall and turned in a panic to Jerry, "We have to leave." Jerry knew if he wanted to keep seeing me he couldn't be late getting me home. We left.

I never did know how that movie ended.

We parked in front of my house with only a few minutes to spare.

"Jerry, it's ten. I have to go in now," I pleaded as he nuzzled my neck, seeking one more kiss before exiting the car.

"I know." His lips traveled to my ear. My breath quickened.

"Really, I have to go. I'm so sorry. I wanted to see the end of the movie too. It's not fair, having to leave every movie before it's over," I pouted.

"I agree." His warm breath traveled down the back of my neck.

His next kiss began soft and tender, then became urgent, making me feel all weak. I felt his hand moving up my rib cage, into forbidden territory. Instantly pushing his wandering hand down—again, wanting it to linger, to let him touch me, I managed to whisper, "Walk me up to the door."

With a sigh, Jerry exited and came around the car, but before he opened my door, the porch light blinked: On. Off. On. Off. That was Mom's signal that I had better get in that house in a hurry. I knew that if I didn't, I would be grounded. And the Senior Prom was coming up.

Mom gave me the third-degree many times, in an accusatory tone of voice, asking about what we had been doing on our dates. Grilling by the local sheriff might have been tougher, but not as thorough. I'm not sure where Mom's fear of premarital sex ranked, but it lurked right up there with her fear of the dark and swimming. I once thought it was because of her puritanical upbringing, but decades later decided it may have been based on her own intense sexual drive, especially when all her senses were zinging.

When it came to sex education, you would think that a doctor and a nurse would be able to handle it. Dad left it up to Mom and she botched it. When I turned fifteen Mom handed me a small book. With a hushed tone and embarrassed look, she said, "Read this, and if you have any questions, come and ask me." The book started with the birds and progressed to the bees. It didn't even have anything about humans in it. That didn't matter. By the time she gave it to me, having pooled plenty of misinformation from my friends and Gracie, I already knew the basic details.

What I didn't know was what to do if I ever encountered a child molester. Both parents should have explained to me at an earlier age what that entailed and what to do if it happened.

When eleven, I desperately needed someone to help me cope with a horrible experience. I started to tell Mom during the time we spent together in the hospital in Dallas, but the words wouldn't come out of my mouth. Especially since I knew she would blame me.

Teen Angst: Confrontation # 1

About a month before my surgery, I went to spend the night with a friend whose mother was gone for the evening. As I walked in the door my friend said, "Daddy is going to teach us how to dance." She put on some slow dance records and insisted that both of us dance with him at the same time. She stood next to him and I stood behind her. He put his arms around her and his hands on my sides, under my arms that were raised to hold onto his forearms. We three were awkwardly moving to the music when his hands moved down and his thumbs brushed over my budding breasts. I stumbled.

What is he doing? That must have been an accident, I thought.

He did it again.

I stopped dancing, embarrassed, frightened, confused about what to do.

"Diane, why won't you dance with us? Come on. Dance." My friend begged and begged me. I refused, head down, afraid to look at her creepy daddy.

Early the next morning, standing in their only bathroom with the door open, I peered into the mirror over the sink trying to put my lip gloss on straight.

He entered behind me, reached out, put his hands around me and started fondling my tiny breasts.

I froze, staring at his ugly, leering, grinning face in the mirror.

Then I got mad. Hitting his hands away, I declared, "I'm going to tell Mrs. X if you don't stop touching me. " He stopped, just as his daughter, my friend, walked in. She heard what I said.

To cover up his sick, disgusting behavior, he acted like he tried to interfere with my lip gloss by putting his horrible finger on my lips. Ugh.

"Oh Daddy, stop bothering her," my friend said.

Sitting at their kitchen table, my friend's mother kept chattering away, asking why I wasn't eating. Even water wouldn't go past the lump in my throat. Close to tears, not looking at him, or at her, or my friend, I managed to mumble that I didn't eat breakfast.

Like most children who are molested, I became too scared, too upset and too ashamed to tell anyone, even Gracie. I felt guilty, dirty, like I was the one who had done something wrong. I knew Mom would blame me. So I didn't tell, even though I awakened, frozen in fear, seeing his leering grin in that mirror again and again.

I did feel a moment of triumph when I told him to stop. Standing up for myself felt scary, but powerful.

Mom's love of shopping at the beginning of a spell became legendary just before Gracie started her senior year. Mom came into the kitchen as Gracie and I were munching on some peanut butter and cracker snacks after school. With a huge grin and impish look she said, "Your dad is always surprising us by bringing home a new car. Let's surprise him. Come on, let's go buy a car."

And did we ever.

Walking into the show room, we three females scanned the six cars on display and instantly, three sets of feet headed for the cutest, the most exciting, the snazziest blue and white Ford convertible ever made—fabulous beyond my wildest dreams. Thirty minutes later, Mom's boring sedan traded in, she floored the gas pedal and grinning from ear to ear with hair wildly blowing, we flew all the way home.

She surprised Dad all right.

What a lark. Having a Mom whose spells included wild spending sprees did have its perks.

Spell, or no spell, my lack of personal spending money remained subject to Mom's financial mismanagement. Her fear of being alone after dark became her reason for not allowing Gracie or me to babysit at night, the main paying job available to teens in our town. Thus, when my friends and I stopped at the Dairy Queen, I listened as they ordered hamburgers, cokes, fries and shakes. I would order the cheapest item offered—a lime-ice. I loved the tart-salty taste and crunchy texture anyway. Chomping slowly, I could sometimes make it last as long as their hamburgers.

Mom's lack of money growing up—and her quirky spells—led her to spend erratically as an adult. Not having discretionary money when young had the opposite effect on me. To this day my fear of being broke always hovers in the background.

Mom had an interesting way of getting things she wanted.

One night in December while we sat around the dinner table, she remarked "I don't want a mink stole. Jessie's and Tillie's are beautiful. But I don't need one."

A week later she commented in Dad's presence, "Annie's mink stole is lovely, but I don't need one."

Later that day Dad paused in the utility room doorway watching me wrap Christmas presents at a card table. Rolls of bright Christmas paper and spools of ribbon were piled high on the sewing machine. Shiny, wrapped boxes covered the tops of the washer and dryer.

"What are you getting Mom for Christmas?" I asked him.

"I don't know. What does she want?"

"A mink stole."

"But she has said over and over that she doesn't want a mink stole," he said with a puzzled look on his face.

"That's because she does."

Clued in to her double-talk, he bought her one. She adored her new fur—and Dad for giving it to her.

Their relationship certainly had serious challenges, but that first spark of love never died. As critical as she was of me, I never once heard her criticize my Dad—not to his face, or to anyone else.

WHEN GRACIE LEFT FOR COLLEGE, things changed around the house. Gone was the two-against-one ratio with Mom. So I did what experience had taught me was safest. I vanished from her life. We lived in the same house, but not together. I appeared at mealtimes and to do my Responsibilities, but otherwise I stayed out of her sight, wondering how I could survive another spell, how I could stand the remaining months until I left for college—or Prince Charming showed up.

8

Escaping from Mom

ONE SUNDAY MORNING NEAR THE end of my senior year in high school, I was sitting in the balcony of the First Baptist Church and caught a good looking guy looking at me. He grinned. I grinned back. We kept making eye-contact all during that Sunday's sermon. Dawdling on my way to the car after the service, I wasn't surprised when he came right up and introduced himself.

Tony turned out to be a student pilot at the nearby air force base. It only took a few seconds for this six foot tall, sandy haired man with the blue eyes, chiseled Roman nose and rakish grin to captivate me. We had just started to chat when Mom approached the car. Noticing her, Tony introduced himself.

"I'm Mrs. Dweller, Diane's mother," she responded, checking him out, up and down.

"This is your mother?" His shocked voice indicated she looked much too young to be my mother.

"Yes, I am," she said with a coquettish smile and lilting voice. "I hope we see you again next Sunday."

He had charmed us both.

THE NEXT WEEK AT SCHOOL I was selected to represent the town as the Armed Forces Day Queen at the local air force base. Arriving for the festivities the following Saturday, I was surprised to discover my escort for the day of special events would be none other than Tony.

He explained, "They asked if anyone knew you. When I said I did, some of my buddies thought I was kidding."

During the hours together I learned he was twenty-five years old, a

Escaping from Mom

successful football quarterback and a college graduate—a giant step up from the local high school boys. By the end of that day I was smitten as only a seventeen-year-old girl can be—with one hundred percent of every ounce of my being.

We had a fun-filled whirlwind romance over the next three months, seeing each other as often as his training and Mom allowed. Each date, I all but pinched myself that this dashing college graduate could be interested in me, a high school senior.

ONE NIGHT AT THE END of the summer, two weeks before Tony left for further pilot training in Phoenix, we were in the back yard, peering up at the clear night sky trying to identify constellations when he took me in his arms. A warm breeze and the fragrance of Mom's roses wafted around us. Looking steadily into my eyes, he tenderly whispered those three magic words I had dreamed of hearing all my life, "I love you." Followed by, "I've never felt this way about anybody, ever."

"I love you too," I said, feeling goose-bumps travel down my arms. He kissed my cheek, the tip of my nose and then my lips, a long lingering but tender kiss. The pulse pounding in my ears all but blocked out his next sentence. I thought he said the M word. Had I heard him right? Did he just say, "I want to marry you?"

"YES."

Incredible. Tony wants to marry me. He loves and wants to marry ME.

I ARRANGED FOR US TO meet with Mom and Dad the next night. Tony and I sat on the rattan love seat in the den across from them, holding increasingly damp hands. I beamed while listening as Tony, proclaiming his love for me, asked my parents for my hand in marriage. Marriage. The ultimate escape. The huge grin across my face started to make my cheeks hurt.

Expecting this pronouncement, Mom and Dad had their response ready. "Diane's so young and we want her to get a good start on a college education. We want you to wait two years."

Two years? I didn't want to wait even two days. We finally agreed to wait one year. I'm sure my parents thought that time and distance would cool our romance.

Tony left for Phoenix to complete his training and get his permanent base assignment.

The next month I packed up my belongings and headed to college with Gracie, excited about escaping Mom at last, but not terribly interested in getting any particular degree. I expected to marry Tony and have children, not a career.

Five weeks into my first college term Asian flu swept through the campus and hit me hard. Ending up in the hospital with double pneumonia, I missed too much class time to catch up that term. What a downer.

Criminals heading to prison probably feel happier, I thought, as I lay in the back seat of the car, hating each mile that took me back home to live with Mom. I had relished the joy and glorious freedom from her constant criticism during the past few weeks. How I would ever adjust to living with her again?

Still recovering two weeks later, I answered the ringing phone and heard Tony's excited voice say these life-changing words, "I got orders for England for three years, and I want to take you with me as my wife." Marriage sounded like much more fun than courses and exams, and I would be living half-way around the world from you-know-who. I instantly said, "Yes."

Mom and Dad were not happy about this change in our plans, but realizing I would be eighteen in a few weeks and free to marry him without their permission, they reluctantly agreed.

In order for me to be on his military travel orders, we needed to be married in the next three weeks. Mom went into high gear planning a home wedding, making most of the decisions without consulting me—a fitting exit scenario. Still weak from my illness, I focused on the exciting reality that I would be leaving home—finally and forever. How far away was England? So far away I envisioned three years without even phone calls from Mom. Giddy with love and the excitement of moving to the romantic land of Sir Lancelot and Guinevere, I lived in a fog of euphoria those three weeks.

I felt jubilant during our wedding, looking into Tony's eyes as he promised to love, honor and cherish me. My imaginary Prince Charming had actually arrived.

WITHIN THREE WEEKS OF OUR arrival in Phoenix, I realized I really didn't know Tony at all. He didn't live up to my expectations of a husband, nor did I as his wife. I expected my husband to do things with me, not go out with the guys and come home vomiting drunk every weekend. This shocked me as I had never seen him take even one sip of one drink, much less get drunk. I also didn't expect him to make crude suggestive comments involving me to his friends—or stand there and demand I pick his clothes up off the floor.

As the early weeks of our marriage passed, Tony's criticisms increased, shaking my wobbly self-confidence even more. Doubts about my ability to be a competent wife, to make him happy, began to erase all the joy I felt earlier. Stunned, I tried and tried to gain Tony's approval. Instead I got more corrections. Everything I did seemed to be wrong.

When I asked, "What have I done wrong?"

His response, "You should know."

SITTING ALONE AT THE FORMICA kitchen table in the breakfast nook in our rented house, I tried to write upbeat thank-you notes for our wedding gifts while my mind whirled. This marriage wasn't starting off well. Confusion about how to do things to please Tony, plus tension and heartbreak every time he criticized me or gave me a disapproving stare, exploded in my head.

Oh God, what have I done? Married my mother?

Survival behavior learned in childhood started surfacing. Withdraw. Don't confront or challenge him. Keep silent. Act like what he said didn't hurt. I became watchful, wary. I tried to make him happy. Often I could not figure out what I did that upset him, I kept telling myself to keep the peace. Try harder. It will work out. You just need to give it time.

STOPPING IN NORTH CREEK ON our way from Phoenix to England, we stayed only one night. The next morning as our car started down the driveway I felt some of the pre-wedding euphoria return. I turned, waved farewell to my parents and said hello to freedom from Mom's criticisms and control. I had escaped from her for good.

We stopped in Arkansas so I could hug Granny goodbye, then headed to Georgia to say goodbye to Tony's parents. It was also a get-acquainted trip for me as I had yet to meet them. Tony's mom turned out to be a tiny lady with a pleasant disposition—a real sweetheart. I didn't take to his dad, a big, burly man, especially after observing his controlling attitude toward his wife.

She wasn't allowed to go anywhere without him. Or even to drive a car. That this dominating man was Tony's example of a husband did not bode well.

Prior to heading to New York to board the military troop ship for England, we stopped in Atlanta. A group of Tony's football buddies threw a party for us in a small, three-room apartment. It started well. I liked his friends but wondered about some of the women. Were they the type he told me about in excruciating personal detail—the type who hung around the jock dorm and provided fabulous free sex to the athletes, including him?

Tony left me on my own as he partied and reminisced with his friends. The throb of rock rhythms pulsed the air, the booze flowed freely, the voices got louder. Chatting with others I suddenly realized Tony hadn't been in the living room for a while. I looked in the kitchen. Nope. No sign of him. That left only one room—the bedroom—and someone had shut that door. As I moved toward the bedroom door I heard someone say, "Uh-oh." Dread began to flow through me. A snare drum started beating in my chest.

Trembling, I reached for the door knob, afraid of what I would see on the other side. I paused, took a shallow gasp of air and slowly pushed the door open. There sat my husband, as close as possible, to one of the bimbos—on the bed in the closed bedroom. She looked at me, then at him. Realizing I must be the wife or the girlfriend, she made a hasty exit. Tony looked guilty. Real guilty. Like he had been caught in the act. They were still dressed, but it was obvious I had interrupted something he should not have been doing. They weren't "just talking" as he instantly claimed. I wasn't that gullible.

It had been only six weeks since he lovingly looked in my eyes and pledged to forsake all others and cleave only unto me. My body, my mind went numb. Turning, I made a hasty exit from the party, feeling betrayed. Out on the street, I looked for a taxi, not sure where I was or where to go. Not a cab in sight.

How could he? Who was this man, my husband? What if I had opened the door faster? What was he doing to look so guilty? Pain shot through me as my trust in Tony cracked. Anger erupted. Not just at him but at myself. I felt stupid. Real stupid. I had made a huge mistake.

I started walking down the street. Tony came after me, grabbing my arm. We left the party. The silence between us on the way back to the motel pulsated with tension. My options? Go to England and try to make it work or go back home and admit I had made a mistake to you-know-who.

We sailed for England on New Year's Day, a holiday I would come to dread.

RENTING A HOUSE NEAR BENTWATERS Air Force Base, located northeast of London, presented a challenge. We ended up staying in a drafty hotel on the North Sea coast several weeks while looking for suitable housing. The wind whistled around the windows of our large room, making the heavy, damask drapes sway. With each sway, an icy breeze circled the room. The only heat source—a small, metered, two-bar electric heater—required a two shilling piece every fifteen minutes. Shivering, my nighttime attire expanded to include not only a nightgown, but a robe, wooly socks, gloves and a knit hat.

When Tony and I arrived back at the hotel one night, four weeks after we moved in, he peered around suspiciously and whispered, "Come on. Hurry. We have to go up the backstairs."

"Why are we going this way?"

"Shhhh. She'll hear you," he responded, acting all secretive and excited.

I followed quietly. Once in the room, I quizzed him. "Why did we sneak up the back stairs?"

"I haven't paid the bill," he confessed with a grin.

"Why not? Don't we have the money?" I asked, suddenly worried that we must be broke. Tony controlled our finances.

"Sure, we have it. It's just fun to see how long I can go without paying it."

Not pay the bill? Fun? What kind of ethics did my husband have? What kind of man doesn't pay his bills? Or thinks it is fun to sneak around, hiding from the manager? Why is he doing this? For the excitement? My dad always paid his bills. Even Mom paid hers.

Two weeks later when I started to move our belongings out, the manager called me into her crowded office. She stared at me, frowning. "You need to settle the bill. We have not been paid since the second week." I sat down, stunned, humiliated, feeling my face flush. Tony had gone to work without paying, even though he knew we were moving out today. He left me to face the consequences of his actions.

I sat there, hand poised over the check, realizing with a sinking feeling that I married a man who got excited about breaking all types of rules.

Signing the check, I could only hope we had enough money to cover it.

I moved our belongings into a tiny, quaint English cottage twenty minutes from the base. Over sixty years old, the drafty bungalow had only four electrical outlets in the whole place—and no furnace, just portable heaters that didn't do the job. Teeth chattering, I chose daily to wear wool pants over long johns and double sweaters—inside the house. We finally bought a large kerosene heater and managed to keep one room heated to all of a toasty sixty degrees.

The kitchen, an add-on, was so tiny I could squat in one spot and sweep the whole room with a hand broom. The British version of a refrigerator in the 1950s consisted of a cupboard with an opening to the frigid outside air to keep daily purchases from spoiling. We purchased a real fridge but it had to be put in the dining room. We also bought a small not-fully-automatic clothes washing machine that reduced the kitchen space even more.

I set about making curtains and turning the cottage into a home. Tony started his job at the base, flying almost daily. He sometimes had alert duty that kept him at the base all night. In the middle of the Cold War, planes stayed constantly loaded with nuclear bombs with crews on standby, ready to take off instantly. Tony's secret target was somewhere in Russia, so far that he wouldn't have enough fuel to get back to England.

Frequent anti-American Ban-the-Bomb marches in England started getting rowdy. On the days they were held, phone relays warned the American wives. We were not to leave our homes that day. If war started, I had to be ready for another wife and her four children, who lived on the base, to come to stay with me in our tiny bungalow.

Times were tense enough without having a tense marriage.

I MISSED GRACIE'S BEAUTIFUL WEDDING. She married her college sweetheart that June. Pictures of the event finally came via ship eight weeks later. Few people or letters flew across the pond in the Fifties. The pictures were preceded by a colorful, descriptive letter from Gracie. I could just envision the following scene she described.

Mom, Dad and Gracie were to arrive at the church by 7:15, so at seven o'clock, Gracie, in her beautiful long lace wedding gown and train climbed into the back seat of the car. Dad got in the driver's seat. At 7:05 he honked the horn. At 7:10 he got out to go find Mom. Repeated calls got no response. Finally he spied her outside bending over the flower beds doing something in her mother-of-the-bride dress and stocking feet.

"What are you doing? We have to leave. We're going to be late."

"I'm putting some blooms in the spots where these plants didn't bloom. Hand me those last two coke bottles with the blooms in them."

"People are not going to notice a few missing blooms during the reception," he said, handing her the coke bottles. Ignoring him, she bent over, dug a hole with a garden trowel and stuck another bottle in the ground.

"Yes they are," she insisted, grunting as she bent over again. "There. That's the last one. Oh dear, I've got a run in my hose. I have to change. Go tell Gracie I'm coming."

I EAGERLY LOOKED FORWARD TO Tony bringing the mail home each evening. Letters from home, even from Mom, were bright spots in the dreary British winter when the sun, if it shone at all, appeared after nine in the morning and disappeared before five in the afternoon. I missed my Texas sunshine. Mom wrote often and I could tell she was hyper when her letters contained cryptic, disjointed sentences that wandered all over the pages. Gracie wrote that Mom still had spells and fender-benders, making me happy to be so far away.

My letters home focused on the quaintness of England, the narrow streets, the number of vintage cars, shopping at the ironmongers and green grocers. And how at the end of each movie the audience stood during the playing of the British national anthem while watching a scene of Queen Elizabeth riding a horse. Never did I give anyone a hint of the turmoil in my marriage.

My marriage certainly was not what I expected. Our social life revolved around events at the Officer's Club where drinking to excess was the norm. Driving a drunk husband home, party after party, got old, real fast. Though perplexed over the unpaid bill, his questionable actions with the girl on the bed and his drinking, I remained determined to do everything I could to make my marriage work, and to make Tony glad he had married me, to make him want only me, and no one else. I tried hard to please him.

I didn't.

People wonder why women who are verbally abused by a controlling husband don't stand up to them or leave. I learned why, the hard way. At first you are shocked that the loving, tender man you married is berating you. Surely he will change back to the terrific guy you dated. You want to please him, trying first one thing and then another. But it only takes another criticism, scowl or a day of his silent treatment to know you didn't. You try harder to do the right thing. The right way. His way. Another irritated look. You fail. Again. And again. Repeat this daily, weekly for six months and it is the happy bride who changes. She begins to believe what he tells her. It is her fault.

When a child, I longed to be held and hear these words: "I love you. You're pretty. You're wonderful. You can do it." It didn't happen. I had a mother and now a husband whose main communication with me focused on the negative, on everything I did wrong. Once again the question swirled around my mind: Why am I so unlovable? Once again I felt totally incompetent and incapable of ever doing anything right.

How incapable, I learned scowl by scowl. As the months went by and Tony's verbal criticisms or silent treatment continued, I became fearful, afraid I would do something that he didn't like and see that look of irritation flash across his face. When we were with other people, if Tony stood in earshot, I shut my mouth and didn't say a word. My old friend Tension became my constant companion each time Tony came near in public. My shattered self-confidence decreased as my fear of displeasing Tony increased.

"I don't like the way you hold your hands. Don't do it anymore," Tony exclaimed one evening driving home from an event at the base. I didn't know what he meant until the next week when we again went to the Officer's Club. I stood in a group of friends enjoying the conversation until Tony joined the circle. He took one look at me, reached over and SLAP. He hit my hand, held loosely over my slightly enlarged pregnant abdomen. The sound echoed. All talking and laughing in the group ceased as people looked from me to him and back. Humiliated, I looked down, tears welling in my eyes.

After that, I not only stopped talking in public, I kept my hands down at my sides. I reverted to behavior learned as a child—become invisible, keep-the-peace, keep silent, don't make her/him mad. Mom had trained me well on how to respond to a critical, controlling husband.

'Make it work' became my mantra. I still desperately tried to please him. My question, "What do you want me to do differently" always got the silent stare, or, "You should know." Trying to figure out my misdeeds, without explicit clues, led to misguided actions that irritated him more. I stayed trapped in an unending loop of failing, without clues as to how or why.

Escaping from Mom 93

And I was about to become a mother. Would I fail at that too?

Having told my family we expected this baby on Halloween, by October 31st everyone assumed labor would start any minute. One week passed. Ten days. Still no labor. Sunday, the day I reached fourteen overdue days, the phone rang. "Hello Diane, It's your mother. I just had to call even if it is expensive." Twenty questions followed including, "May I talk to Tony now?"

"He's not here right now. He'll be so sorry he missed your call." I didn't tell her he was in France, coaching the football team from our base. Or that I was alone and scared. Beyond scared. Convinced-I-might-die-in-childbirth-scared.

Tony did return in time for his son's birth in mid-November, sixteen days late.

IN ENGLAND, DURING THE FIFTIES, birthing included a ten-day stay in the British hospital. On day ten, eager to get home, I had myself and baby Alex ready half an hour before the agreed upon time Tony would come get us that morning. Eleven o'clock came and went. Eleven thirty. Twelve. He didn't answer the phone. Alex began crying, wanting to nurse. I tried to soothe him, hoping his daddy would arrive any minute. It didn't work. I fed Alex, constantly afraid Tony would arrive and be mad because we weren't ready. Twelve thirty. I nibbled at my lunch. Finally at two o'clock Tony arrived.

"Why are you three hours late?" I asked.

"I told you I would be here at two o'clock. You didn't listen to me."

Yeah, like "two o'clock" sounded like "eleven o'clock." I knew I hadn't heard it wrong. What could have kept him? His challenging stare lingered too long, making me suspicious he was lying. Why would he lie? In my postpartum hormone-reversal state I couldn't cope with the most obvious reason, so I went silent and emotionally numb, a familiar state of being.

I LOVED BEING A MOTHER. Alex turned out to be a placid baby and in the next six weeks we settled into our routine, bonding more with each precious moment. I adored him and he seemed to like me fine. He had very few complaints. Of course the laundry tripled with our new addition, especially with the terrycloth nappies that the Brits used for diapers.

"You better not be washing those diapers in the washing machine." Tony declared.

"Why?" I stared at him, stunned at this new order.

"You're washing my clothes in there and you are not to wash any diapers in there too."

"Oh, of course not." I acquiesced.

No diapers in the washing machine? Was he crazy? Where did he expect me to hand wash the diapers? In the bath tub or the kitchen sink? A backlog of rebellion stirred deep within me.

Women who fear openly rebelling against controlling husbands find more subtle ways. Later that day, the scent of revenge filled the air as I dumped the pail of soiled diapers directly on top of his shirts in the washing machine.

A smug got-ya feeling resurfaced every time he put on one of his diaper-clean shirts.

In December I thought things were going better in our marriage until New Year's Eve. Attending the gala in the connected Quonset huts used as the Officer's Club, we danced and socialized waiting for the magic stroke of midnight. As the countdown began, I started looking for Tony. Not in the ballroom. Not in the bar. Or the game room. Midnight came and went. Still no sign of him. Not inside or out. The car still sat where we parked it. I kept searching the facility. No sign of him. Finally, twenty-five minutes later, he appeared in the ballroom.

"Where have you been?" I asked in a more demanding tone than I had ever used with him.

"I've been here. Where were you?" He starred directly in my eyes, challenging me to dispute that obvious lie.

"Looking for you."

"Well, now you found me," he declared.

Twenty-five minutes. Missing for twenty-five minutes. I knew now, in my collapsing heart, he was probably with another woman. Who? How long had it been going on?

If I had proof . . . thoughts of leaving Tony had darted through my mind more than once, but being Southern Baptist, I found the idea of divorce abhorrent, especially in the Fifties when divorces were considered taboo and divorcees wanton women. While I had made a bad decision, I was determined to succeed in my marriage, especially with a baby. I had to make it work.

9

Cold Anger:
Confrontation # 2

A WEEK AFTER THE NEW YEAR'S party, Tony arrived home from the base one evening very excited and in a hurry. He threw the mail on the dining table, hustled to change his clothes and headed toward the door yelling, "I forgot to tell you I have to officiate a basketball game at the base gym."

Silence settled throughout the house, the baby and puppy both asleep. I took the quiet moments to sit down at the dining table and sort through the mail. A bill. A letter from a friend. The third item startled me. A personal letter to my husband was addressed in girlish script. The return address held only one word—Angel. My gut responded. It knew without a doubt there could only be one reason someone named Angel would be writing my husband. I stared at the envelope for several minutes, dread seeping into every pore. I finally ripped open the flap and pulled out three pages. Torrents of deep, everlasting love flew off the page followed by descriptions of how romantic their stay at the Angel Inn had been. I felt lightheaded as the passionate details of their affair were revealed. Obviously they had been seeing each other for months. I had trouble breathing, reading details no wife wants to know.

What should I do? Was he with her right now? He must have been with her during the New Year Eve's party. And the night before his late arrival at the hospital. His frequent evening trips back to the base to officiate sports became nights of lovemaking between my husband and this English girl in my mind.

I looked for a place to hide that traitorous letter and finally placed it under a drawer in the bedroom vanity. When Tony came home four hours later I feigned sleep. For five fretful days and sleepless nights I pondered what to do. Should I confront him? Should I go to the chaplain at the base for help? Should I take our son and go back to Texas? I felt totally disconnected to reality, as if I were viewing my life through the wrong end of a spyglass.

The wimp in me toyed with the idea of getting on a plane with Alex and disappearing without confronting Tony. I would just leave that awful letter for him to find. Then I imagined going back to Texas, admitting I made a mistake and having to live with Mom—with a baby. Visions of returning to her control under these circumstances quickly dispelled that idea. I knew who she would blame for the failure of my marriage. At nineteen I had no job skills, no education with which to support myself, especially with a newborn. Bewildered, I saw no viable solution.

Tony obviously did not love me anymore. The total love I felt when we married, cracking for months, now crumbled apart. Trust had been broken, beyond repair. Yet a small part of me still yearned for a happy marriage, especially now that we had a child.

I finally got up the nerve to confront him. He walked in the house and started to change out of his uniform. I entered our bedroom, my voice and knees shaky, and said, "You spent the night with an English girl while I was in the hospital after giving birth to our son."

Tony's eyes widened. "What are you talking about?"

"I'm talking about the night you spent in the Angel Inn with another woman. I have a letter to prove it. She wrote you all about it, how much she loves you. And how thrilled she is that you love her."

Blank faced for only a moment, his face transformed into a scowl. "Where is that letter? Give it to me. RIGHT NOW."

I refused, over and over. The fury in his voice escalated, scaring me. Frightened by his wrath, I produced the letter. He read it.

"You are stupid to believe this pack of lies." He started berating me for believing it. "She's lying."

I knew who was lying.

Two strained days passed before I got up the courage to say, "I don't believe you."

He retaliated, "I didn't do what she said, but if I did have an affair it would be your fault."

"My fault? How would it be my fault?"

"You should know."

Cold Anger: Confrontation # 2

Was it my fault? Was I a total failure as a wife? A woman? Since childhood, I had been programmed to accept negative comments as true. I, an incompetent child, had turned into an incompetent wife, the reason my husband had to have an affair.

Even if I were to blame, I didn't want to stay married to someone who didn't love me and treated me this way. While life with Mom was negative, this was worse. Since my pre-teens Mom made my shortcomings clear, always telling me exactly what I had done wrong or failed to do. With Tony, it remained a confusing guessing game.

The next morning, bundling us both up, I tucked Alex into his stroller and went for a walk along the quay, seeking solace in nature. Watching the gulls soaring up on the air currents, listening to their cries, I started to cry too. But the gentle sound of the sea as the incoming waves foamed across the rocky shore soon became rhythmically soothing. Looking reality in the eye, weighing my limited options, I decided what I must do.

That night, after removing the dinner dishes from the table, I stood there, steeling myself. Taking several deep breaths I looked at Tony and declared, "I'm leaving. Alex and I are going back to Texas."

Tony looked up at me in disbelief, "What?"

"We are leaving you."

He appeared dumbstruck. Then his reaction totally confused me. Taking me in his arms he started urging me, "Stay. I would never be unfaithful to you. I promise. I'm sorry she wrote that letter. I love you. I love Alex."

Over the next two days the critical, dictatorial Tony disappeared. The charismatic man I fell in love with showed up again, loving and caring, wooing me, "Don't leave, don't leave," he begged.

Had he dumped his English girlfriend? Did he only want a forbidden woman? Her, now me, since I presented a new challenge by threatening to leave?

I didn't believe him, the letter had been too explicit. But after days of vacillation, with a small hope that he would not be unfaithful again, I stayed, praying I wasn't making another huge mistake.

After this confrontation we did have two fairly good years of marriage. Tony appeared to be faithful, or at least much more discreet. Even his criticisms became less harsh, less often. We went on a tour of Europe, to

Paris, Rome, Venice and the Alps. Back in England we went to London for a weekend to see a performance of *My Fair Lady* with the original cast. And we both adored our son, the source of much joy as we watched him learn to crawl, walk, then feed himself, sometimes even finding his mouth on the first try. We did have some fun times and my hopes for a stable marriage soared.

ANOTHER BRIGHT SPOT IN THOSE three years in England came from getting to take art lessons from Cor Visser, a Dutch artist whose watercolors hang in many European museums today. He taught me to see what I was looking at and to draw it accurately—before ever picking up a paint brush. My latent talents blossomed under his guidance and I looked forward to continuing my painting, wherever life took us.

UPON RETURNING TO THE STATES at the end of Tony's three-year military tour, he started looking for a job. After a couple of months of no job offers, he decided to accept my Dad's offer to come back to North Creek and become an assistant administrator for his clinic. This dismayed me, but pregnant again, we had an immediate need for an income and insurance. So back to the lioness's den I went.

The landscape in Texas looked bleak and desolate to me after the lushness of England. The wind still blew daily, worse than I recalled. We rented a small house with a dirt yard. Tony went to work and I started making our rented house into a home complete with a nursery for our new baby.

Three months after our move, my first labor pain hit hard in the middle of the night. The next few progressed rapidly. Tony took me to the hospital before taking Alex over to Mom and Dad's. By the time he arrived back at the hospital with Mom in tow, I was in heavy labor with hard, long contractions occurring constantly. It had only been one hour since the first contraction. This baby, again two weeks late, was finally in a hurry to get here.

Practicing the natural childbirth techniques I learned in England, I focused on my breathing and relaxing one part of my body at a time. Then I heard Mom's voice, "Diane, Diane, here, let me brush your hair," Her comment broke my concentration. I tried to regain my rhythm as I felt the brush sweep through my hair.

Cold Anger: Confrontation # 2

Focus. Focus on breathing. Ignore her. Relax your forehead. Breathe. Relax your mouth. Breathe. Relax . . .

"Open your eyes. Put on this lipstick," she demanded, holding an open tube out to me. "You look too pale."

She totally disrupted my focus just as a massive contraction peaked. I was in transition.

Furious at her stupid lipstick request, I wanted to scream at her at the top of my lungs, *GET OUT OF HERE*, but I knew tensing any of my body would increase the pain. So instead of yelling at her, the most tactful moment of my entire life occurred. I breathed in, blew out. I relaxed my mouth and managed to quietly say, "Please Mom, leave. Leave—me—alone."

Followed by, "Go get the doctor. NOW. I'm pushing."

My precious daughter Andrea arrived before my doctor got his scrub suit on—or I any lipstick.

WE SETTLED INTO LIFE IN North Creek as a family of four, buying our first house. I really enjoyed decorating and set about turning this updated vintage house into a home. It had thick adobe walls. The huge front room that spanned the width of the house included the open areas of the living, dining, kitchen and breakfast rooms. The walls were a soft pale green, the floor was beige brick in a chevron pattern.

The den became my favorite room. One red brick wall held a huge wood-burning fireplace. Southern windows kept the room light and airy and looked out on the terraced patio where the children could play. Our Danish modern teak furniture, brought back from Europe, fit beautifully. This became the room everyone gravitated to.

Our backyard had a Cold War bomb shelter buried in it. Lifting the heavy, lead-lined door, I went down in it. It felt cool, but tomblike. Thinking I should stock it in case of a tornado, I took some bedding, a jug of water and some diapers down there—just in case.

It turned out that life in North Creek was not to be so bad after all. Many of my friends still lived there, so I slid right into an active social life with other young mothers. Tony, the charismatic version, made friends easily, especially with other golfers or hunters. Our married life together, while not joyous, became pleasant.

Seeing busy Mom only a couple of times each week turned out to be less of a problem than I had anticipated. She did continue to have spells periodically. During these turbulent weeks, her insight into what others thought of her, or said, continued to be misread or misconstrued. She thought everyone loved her, that she was the best, the smartest, the most competent. She consistently exhibited an inability to pick up on nonverbal signals from the many people who obviously thought otherwise.

Tony could not stand her. Sunday lunch with my parents after church turned into a period of excruciating emotional stress for me. Tony would sit, eat, then leave to go play golf without saying more than about ten words. Dad picked up on it. Motor-mouth Mom never did.

About the time baby Andrea started toddling, Tony stopped criticizing me. That was because he totally stopped talking to me.

"What have I done wrong now? Why aren't you speaking to me?" I asked several times over the next few days.

No response. He totally ignored me. I had evidently done something very wrong. But what? This was the start of a long period of cold, distant treatment.

One evening he came home from work, walked in the door and past me with no acknowledgment that I stood there. That I even existed. He sent neither his cold stare nor his angry frown in my direction.

"Dinner's almost ready," I called out as he headed to the bedroom. A few minutes later he came back into the living room wearing a different set of clothes. Walking toward the front door, he passed me, a foot away, still ignoring the fact that I stood there.

"Where are you going?"

No response. No glance. A chill traversed my body. I no longer existed.

The door shut behind him. Alex ran to the window and watched his daddy drive away.

I stood there, rooted to the spot, feeling the last flicker of self-worth I had disappear.

Which felt worse: being criticized or being ignored? Mom had done a great job, robbing me of self-confidence through constant criticism. Tony's coldness completed what Mom started. My feeling of being a failure sunk

Cold Anger: Confrontation # 2

to new depths as the holidays passed, filled with long silences between us.

Then on New Year's Day Tony surprised me by asking, "How about going out to La Cantina's for dinner tonight? Can you get a babysitter?

Wow, a date. A night out together. I wondered what prompted this thaw, this attention. Had I been punished enough?

As I got dressed, I glanced in the mirror, pleased to see the pregnancy pooch had finally disappeared. Had Tony noticed?

On the way to the restaurant, I voiced a couple of comments about the children. He even answered. My hopes for a pleasant dinner soared.

Steamy plates of enchiladas, beans and rice were placed before us. I blew on my first bite of enchilada, placed it in my mouth and started to savor the rich, spicy flavor when Tony announced, "I want a divorce."

I looked at my plate. This was not happening. He did not just say he wanted a divorce. The bite of food felt huge. I couldn't swallow. I couldn't say anything. I couldn't breathe. He leaned toward me.

"Did you hear me? I want a divorce," he hissed, glancing at the other tables.

Tears stung my eyes making my plate appear a blurry mess—like my life. I knew he didn't love me anymore. Nor I him. But I thought we would stay married. We had two children, one still a baby. Blinking back tears, refusing to look at him, I lurched up, made my way through the busy tables, out of the restaurant to the car. I still could not swallow that bite. I spit it out.

How could he? How could he ask me for a divorce in a crowded restaurant? Did he think I would sit there and not react in such a public place?

Yes Stupid, he did. Years of my silent acceptance of his demands would make him think I would sit there and do and say nothing but, "Yes."

Shortly, Tony stormed out, got in the car and started in on how I had humiliated him by walking out.

I didn't listen. I withdrew. I wasn't there. This wasn't happening. But it was.

He moved out.

Mother was mortified. Her daughter, separated from her husband. What would people say?

As the weeks of separation lengthened, I began to start experiencing what life was like when the pendulum stopped swinging through the pit of my marriage. What a relief. No more disgusted looks, no more trying to figure out what I had done wrong. I didn't have to try to please, to placate Tony anymore. Wow. This single life felt pretty good. Except for becoming a divorcee. Except for becoming a single mother with no job and no job skills. And no self-confidence.

Every contact with Mom after the separation started with this litany: "This is terrible. This is awful. You can't get divorced. People are talking about you. What happened? What did you do wrong? I'm so embarrassed. How could you let your marriage fail? What did you do?"

What had I done? Simply tried everything I could to make my marriage a happy one, or to at least stay married. I shook my head, ignoring her questions, too heartsick to answer.

I tried to confide in Dad, knowing I could count on him in a crisis, but some of the details, like how Tony ignored me, were too painful for him to hear. It must have been hard for him to go to work each day and see the person who hurt me so deeply. As the weeks passed, Dad began stopping by my house more often, giving me an extra hug or two. Having at least one parent who didn't berate me really helped.

Gracie, now a homemaker and mother called often, voicing her concern and offering help.

Getting a divorce in a small town in the Bible Belt in the Sixties proved traumatic. When I arrived a little late to a coffee, the first guest who saw me said, "Shhhh." All heads turned. Within seconds the entire room fell silent. I stood there. All eyes on me. Condemned. A failure as a wife.

Failure. Maybe I should monogram the letter F on all my clothes.

The town gossips passed along any juicy tidbit, true or not. I heard the Missionary Society at the church had quite a discussion on whether my divorce met Biblical guidelines.

Citing community property laws in Texas, Tony started demanding that I give him half of the college fund Dad had set aside for me. We had used some of it for the down payment on our house. Knowing these funds were all that stood between me and welfare, I resisted Tony's demands. He wasn't used to that. His demands turned ugly. We hired separate attorneys.

When a good friend of mine finally saw that reconciliation wasn't going to happen, she came over one evening. Sitting in the cozy den, she started

Cold Anger: Confrontation # 2

sharing what her husband had told her had been going on for months. Once again blood seemed to drain from my head and heart as she confirmed my suspicions that started when Tony went hunting and forgot to take his shotgun. Not only did he have another girlfriend, he had hired her to work in his office—in my father's clinic. I could just imagine how that sneaky maneuver excited him.

My friend provided details about the places and dates of some of their liaisons.

I also put two plus one together. I had been troubled with what I thought was a female problem for months. Seeking medical help, the infection had defeated the attempts of my doctor to clear it up. He had finally scheduled a gynecological surgical procedure the next week to clear up some scar tissue from birthing that could be inhibiting treatment. Now I recalled his earlier comment, before our separation, that it might help if both marriage partners were treated. This wasn't a female problem; it was an errant husband problem. This infection was a sexually transmitted disease.

After sharing this information with my attorney, he advised me not to confront Tony—yet. I tried to keep from exploding, especially when Tony called daily with ugly demands for the money. For five days I contained my seething until he came over one morning. With an aura of fighter-jock confidence, he demanded the money and started dictating other terms of the divorce settlement.

Sitting in the teal recliner in our den, dark circles around my eyes, physically and emotionally drained from the surgery the day before, I stared at this man I had once considered Prince Charming.

He started to pace and rant at me. "You will give me half of the college fund. Plus half the house sale and one of the cars.

"You can have your car," I replied, "but NO to the house sale and NO to the college fund."

"NO? If you don't agree to do this I'll take you to court," he threatened, confident that I, the wimp, would do anything to avoid a public trial.

"No. You aren't getting my college fund." I said, growing angrier by the second. Unable to contain my pent up fury, I exploded, spewing these words at him, "I know all about your girlfriend."

"What girlfriend? I don't have a girlfriend. You're sick. Delusional."

Anger raged within me. I wanted to tear him apart. To hurt him like he had hurt me.

"You're lying. You and your girlfriend aren't getting any of my money, now or ever," I declared, eyes narrowed, disgust hanging on every word.

"You're making things up. You're mentally ill, unbalanced. You know I can commit you. All I have to do to get you locked up at the mental hospital is tell them how delusional you are. I don't have a girlfriend. It is all in your head. Once you're in the state hospital, I'll have you declared an unfit mother. Then I'll take all the money—and the children."

I reeled back in horror, unable to even breathe. I knew he could get me locked up for two weeks. Other husbands in Texas had. My stomach lurched.

He's threatening to take Alex and Andrea. No. NO. NO. No one is taking my children.

A volcano of churning, hot anger rocked my aching body, ready to explode. I stared in disgust at this man, my husband for five years, while he continued to harangue me, pacing around the room. I started to lash out, to roar at him. But instead, a foreign feeling of cold, steely resolve crept down my entire body. My hands felt cold. My heart colder. I became calm. Dead cold calm. I had never felt so composed, so totally in control.

In a low, slow voice I stated, "Her name is Jo Ann. You hired her to work with you at Dad's clinic. You took her to Roswell, New Mexico on . . . and stayed at . . ." I continued, listing his numerous transgressions with detailed data, calmly ending with this emphatic statement: "No, you will not take my children, nor will you get any of the money. Ever."

"Lies, all lies. You're delusional. Sick. I'm taking you to court," he declared, running his hand through his hair.

"Fine. Go right ahead. I'll gladly meet you and your co-defendant Jo Ann there." With a frigid voice, I continued, "But you should let your married friend Ted know I'll be calling him and his girlfriend who went with you to Roswell, as witnesses.

"Where did you get that information?" Anger flushed his face. His eyes darted around the room. He knew I had him.

I lied to him to protect my friend. "I hired a private detective when I got suspicious. You ought to remember to take your shotgun when you go hunting."

He stood there staring at me, silent. Several long moments passed, then his shoulders slumped, his body visibly wilted as he realized his ruse had failed. I had details that would hold up in court. With witnesses—other married, cheating witnesses.

He suddenly switched tactics as he had in England when confronted with my decision to leave. He sank to his knees in front of my chair, begging me to forgive him, to take him back.

Hmmm, fool me twice? No. Not-ever-again. The sight of this groveling, lying, cheating man made me sick. I wondered, how could I have ever loved him? How could I have ever let him treat me the way he had?

Still icy calm, my reply said it all, "Get up. You have exactly fifteen minutes to get the rest of your things out of this house and get out of my life."

"TAKE MY CHILDREN." THOSE THREE words whipped the wimp right out of me. While I didn't have the nerve to stand up for myself, I discovered a raging lioness inside me when my cubs were threatened. I, the coward, the doormat, the peace-at-all-costs gal had fought back. I had not given in. Without alimony (still the law in Texas today) and with only paltry child support, I needed that college money to get some job skills to support my children.

Confronting Tony felt terrific. That tiny inner spark of self-confidence, missing for so long, started to glow again. I liked that feeling. I vowed, never again to let any man control me or put me down. From now on I planned to stand up, not just for my children, but for myself too. I had come too close to being totally destroyed. It felt fabulous to start to feel like me again.

Tony left town with the girlfriend he denied existed. Confirmation that she was with him came from another of my friends, the wife of Tony's insurance agent. She happened to pick up the extension phone when Tony called to ask how to file a claim after they had a wreck in her car in Georgia.

There are some advantages to living in a small town.

MOM CONTINUED TO BLAME ME for the breakup of my marriage. "You should have obeyed your husband, as the head of your house. What did you do to make him leave you?" she asked, her tone full of accusations. I had not confided in her about any of our problems, his earlier unfaithfulness or how he treated me privately. Oblivious to all of the signs, she had thought we were happily married.

She wasn't the only one. The day Tony left town, a friend took me to lunch at the country club were Tony had played golf. Not aware of my marital change, when the waitress came to take our order she said, "We just love your husband. When he walks into the room the whole place lights up." Yes, that was the man I fell in love with. The fun, vivacious man, the one with charisma and charm. The one who never showed me the controlling side of his personality before I said those fateful words, "I do."

Why did he marry me? Why did a twenty-five year old carousing party animal marry a seventeen year old girl who didn't even drink?

Why did I marry him?

Hindsight isn't always 20/20. Looking back, was I just too eager to believe in a real Prince Charming? Too young to see Tony realistically? Too desperate for love? Or too thrilled to get away from Mom?

All of the above?

Had I ever felt loved and appreciated, would I have married so young? One cannot know the counterfactual, but I do know that my goal since early childhood, to get away from Mom, to get far away, did impact my decision.

Marriage had not turned out to be the answer to my quest for love and affection. Now, what options did I have? What could I do? How would I manage? I had plenty of questions about our survival as a family of three. And no answers.

10

Starting Over

I ARRIVED AT THE COURTHOUSE EARLY, wearing my best navy dress and matching high heels, lipstick on straight. You don't want to be late for your wedding—or your divorce.

The large, high-ceilinged courtroom was empty except for the judge, two uniformed court officials, a lady court recorder, my attorney and me. While I wasn't required to be present for my divorce hearing, I needed to see, to hear the end of my marriage. Maybe then I would feel closure—whatever that is.

My children were at their daycare center, my parents out of town. Thank goodness.

One of the men in a tan uniform called out my case number. Standing below the high wooden bench, hoping my jumpy insides weren't evident outside, I looked up, taking in the American and Texas flags. The judge, whose ten strands of comb-over appeared plastered down with Brylcreme, nodded to my attorney. He began summing up the agreement I reached with Tony before he left town. He spoke for about five minutes before stepping back beside me.

Bang. The judge's gavel came down. "Petition accepted. Divorce granted," was all he said. What I heard and felt was:

Bang. A deep, dark, gaping abyss opening at the edge of my feet.

Bang. Take one step forward.

RETURNING TO MY LOVELY HOUSE, I wandered through the rooms that once held our intact family. Rooms full of broken dreams now. My wide gold wedding band? Another piece of jewelry to be tossed in a drawer with other unworn trinkets.

Reality hit hard. I sucked in a breath, Divorced. I'm divorced. A divorcee. I abhor that word.

My weary body slumped down in the recliner in the den. Kicking my high heels off, I leaned back and reviewed my situation for the umpteenth time. Facts: I am twenty-three years old, a divor—no, a formerly married woman—with two small children and no income. What next?

A hint of an "I can do it" spirit lifted my thoughts. Having seen my dire financial situation looming when Tony first asked for a divorce back in January, I had immediately enrolled at the local junior college, choosing secretarial training as the quickest route to a paycheck. My self-confidence felt a tiny boost when I received good grades, but now I doubted the wisdom of that idea. Can I succeed as a secretary? I'm a terrible speller and electric typewriters just help me make mistakes faster. After finishing this term I'll have to get some office job. But will the pay be enough? Panic began to reverse the can-do feeling. Doubts that I could do anything right settled in the pit of my stomach.

MY PERSONAL LIFE WASN'T THE only thing blowing up. The entire world was on the brink of blowing itself up in a nuclear war. Literally. October 13, 1962, President Kennedy announced that the Russians were building nuclear missile sites in communist Cuba. He gave them an ultimatum: remove them or we will. Television announcers broke into every program, giving the latest news in tense voices. Soviet war ships were streaming toward Cuba. Our navy formed a blockade to keep them out. The Russians started working on the missile sites around the clock. Then one of our U2 planes flying over Cuba was shot down. Shouts for retaliation were heard around the country. The war drums started beating. The Cold war turned red hot. Both the clock and the bombs were ticking, ticking.

I restocked our backyard bomb shelter with fresh water and canned food and new flashlights. My active children couldn't understand why I just wanted to sit and hold them.

For thirteen days the world waited for atom bombs to start exploding. Just as it appeared an atomic war was unavoidable, Khrushchev, the Soviet leader, blinked. Their ships turned back.

I turned back to trying to resolve my own crisis.

THE NEXT WEEK ANDREA, NOW one, and three-year-old Alex and I moved out of our nice home and into a tiny rental house with a sticker-burr-patch for

Starting Over

a yard. My days consisted of attending classes, getting the children to and from daycare, playing with them, cooking dinner, bathing and tucking them in bed, then homework and studying while doing the laundry. Each day: get up and do it all over again. Housework was saved for the weekends. Being this busy meant I didn't have time for poor-me moments, but some did slip in now and then, especially when the children were tired and whiney. I discovered just how hard single parenting and a full-time college schedule could be. Staying calm and collected at the end of exhausting days wasn't easy. I didn't always manage to keep my cool.

Sometime every day, the phone would ring.

"Where have you been? What are you doing?" Mom followed her questions with what she thought I should be doing. I tried to avoid her daily inquisition, especially when I had a rare date, a hard-to-hide occurrence in a small town. Regular dating didn't interest me, nor ever marrying again, but occasional attention from a man gave my shattered ego a huge boost. My focus stayed on getting through this semester, getting a job and making the best life possible for me and my children—solo. No more negative relationships—ever.

Shortly before I completed my second college term, Dad came over one evening after the children were tucked in bed. His solemn expression told me we were going to have a serious talk. We sat down in my tiny living room on the remaining pieces of my teak furniture. Looking me in the eye, he asked, "What are your plans?

"I plan to finish this term and then get the best office job I can."

"Have you considered taking a regular college course and getting a degree?"

Had I ever.

"DAD, I WOULD LOVE TO, but my college fund won't cover tuition, childcare and home expenses for four years." My big Texas-sized child support amount of $200 a month didn't, even in the 1960s, begin to house, feed, clothe and medically care for two children.

He nodded, then said, "I offered you a college education earlier, and you chose marriage. I'll offer it to you one more time and support you and the children until you get a degree—on several conditions."

Wary all of a sudden, I asked, "What conditions?"

Dad leaned forward in his chair, "First, that you finish what you start. I don't want you to get half way through and give up. You weren't the best student in high school."

I stared at him in disbelief. "What do you mean? I had almost a four point grade average—higher than Gracie's. What made you think I wasn't an excellent student?"

He looked down at the linoleum tiled floor of my living room, pondered something for several moments, then shrugged. I knew who had planted that idea.

"What are the other conditions?" I asked, shifting my position to relieve the tension between my shoulders.

"As a single mother, becoming a school teacher is a good idea. You'll have vacation times the same as the children."

I nodded. Even though I didn't want to be a teacher, I recognized that becoming one would be the smart thing to do.

"And, he continued, "I think you should teach English or History. Those teachers are always in demand."

"I'll agree to teach, but may I choose what I teach?" Dad mulled that over and finally nodded. I could see he regretted that nod as soon as I announced I wanted to teach art. The art lessons with Cor Visser in England had awakened my desire to develop the only talent I seemed to have.

With the opportunity to get a college degree, climbing out of my divorce abyss suddenly looked possible. Incredibly grateful for Dad giving me this second chance, I knew I could do it. The alternative? Without his help I might have to become a welfare mother as child care costs would take most of any secretarial wages—the predicament many single mothers find themselves in even today. How fortunate I was to have a dad whose love and generosity ran as deep as the pit I now lived in.

I thrived at the junior college, becoming a diligent student, making the Dean's List, validating Dad's belief in me. After failing at marriage, I rejoiced in every small success—every paper, every test I passed. One barrier from my marriage did emerge in the classroom. Tony had humiliated me so many times in public by correcting what I said, or how I stood or acted, that my habit of becoming invisible in public consisted of never uttering a single word or making any movement to call attention to myself.

One day I entered my English classroom, keeping my head down as I took my seat to avoid eye contact with anyone. The instructor started the class by asking a simple question. Looking down at her seating chart, she called my name. I froze. I knew the answer cold, but all I could do was look down at my desk, my cheeks hot, tears welling as I shook my head, indicating I didn't know.

My self-esteem had been so totally eroded that I, who five years before had relished addressing the entire high school student body, could not even answer a simple question in a junior college class of fifteen younger students. But slowly, one good grade at a time, one successful test after another, one semester after another, I gained the confidence to look up. I finally garnered enough confidence to contribute my thoughts aloud. Good grades and feedback from my professors confirmed I could do something right after all—except in Mom's eyes.

While at her house one afternoon, I overheard her on the phone in the breakfast room telling a friend what she had said as the guest speaker at the Officers Wives Club at the nearby base.

"I spoke about the importance of a woman's role in the home," she said. "I told them we had two daughters. Gracie, our older daughter, was never a problem, an excellent student. She finished college and married her college sweetheart. Now she is a wonderful mother, busy rearing their three children. Both of our daughters had the same parents, the same home and upbringing. We just don't know what went wrong with our other daughter."

Thanks Mom, I really needed that.

DID GRACIE AND I HAVE the same mother? I suspected when Gracie was five years old, Mom's behavior was calmer, more nurturing than when I was the same age. After Mom lost the baby, her screaming and whippings escalated, sending me scared and shaking into hiding. Her scary behavior and tension had reverberated throughout our home until Dad took her to Galveston. Her furious, angry actions toward me during my earliest memories created deep, negative feelings toward her—as a mother to avoid. Twenty years later she could still make me feel unloved with a scowl or critical comment. Like the one she just made to an audience about what a disappointment I am.

MOM WAS NOT THE BABY-SITTING type of granny. Much too busy to do so, she rarely watched my children, especially after the day she lost four-year-old Alex.

At least she honestly reported what happened.

Alex had been helping Mom work on her extensive flower beds in her back yard until she looked up and didn't see him.

"Alex, Alex," she called over and over.

No response. No little brown haired boy anywhere in sight.

She banged on the neighbor's door, "HELP. Help me look. Alex's disappeared. Oh God, where can he be?" Frantic, she and the neighbor searched everywhere.

"I'll call the police," the neighbor said.

An hour later, a fireman spotted Alex between the cedar bushes, climbing the hill behind Mom's house. He had walked three blocks down the street, gone through a huge, busy hospital parking lot and started climbing the hill.

Realizing I could not trust her to maintain attention on the children, even when she wasn't hyper, I ended Mom's rare babysitting help. I should have continued that policy, because three years later, she, who was afraid of the water and couldn't swim, decided to take both children swimming at a private club—without my knowledge or permission.

She confessed, "When we got to the pool, they stopped me at the gate and asked me to show my club membership card. I ransacked my purse and searched in my wallet for several minutes but I couldn't find it, so they had to send someone to the club house to check on my membership. That's when I looked up to check on the children and saw Andrea clinging to the inside edge of the pool in over five feet of water. She scared me to death."

I felt chills and goose bumps travel down my arms. Andrea could have drowned. She didn't know how to swim.

Distracted twice, Mom had lost my son and almost drowned my daughter. Her rare babysitting days were definitely over until the children were older—a lot older—and could not only swim, but use the telephone to call for help.

MOM'S FRIENDS IN OUR SMALL town were very aware of her spells. When a spell occurred, her friends either coped with her antics or ignored her until normal behavior returned. Occasionally her best friend Jessie would tell her, "Dixie, others are talking about you." Unfortunately by the time Jessie got

Starting Over   113

the nerve to say that, Mom was too hyper to care what others thought of her.

Decades later, sitting on Jessie's beautiful antique sofa in her apartment in a retirement home, I asked her, "Jessie, what was it like for you, her friend, when Mom became hyper?"

Jessie let out a big laugh before she described Mom's spells this way: "Dixie could really go on some wing-dingers. It was like she was on roller skates heading downhill. There was just no stopping her."

She shared this example of what Mom did one time: "I planned a luncheon and bridge party for twenty women and invited Dixie to be a guest. I didn't ask her to, but your mom started helping me, changing what I had planned. She even asked the florist what I had ordered for the table centerpieces—and changed the order without consulting me. I didn't know about the change until I stopped to pick up the arrangements the day of the luncheon and saw the different flowers—and the big difference in the bill.

At the club, I put out name cards to show where I wanted each guest to sit, and by whom. Dixie arrived early, took one look at them and started rearranging them to her satisfaction. I was irritated, but I let her. I knew it was useless to try to reason with Dixie during one of her spells. Your mother then proceeded to greet the guests like she was the hostess as they arrived. As the guests were leaving, I heard them thanking Dixie for the lovely party." Jessie laughed and with a shake of her head concluded, "Dixie got the credit. I got the bills."

MOM DID PRODUCE A VARIETY of challenges the last year I lived in North Creek—still spending wildly during spells, backing into things, ignoring feedback, criticizing me, taking over and running her clubs. She appeared to go through life like that cartoon character Mr. Magoo—oblivious to the disaster she left in her wake.

After each of her spells ended, friends and family reacted. Her close friends forgave her any indiscretions. Casual friends who disappeared during the worst times would slowly start to respond to her calls again. Some didn't. Dad would have to fill up her bank account. Gracie and I would try to erase from our memories the criticisms she heaped on us. Being older didn't make her comments to us any less hurtful.

Now that Tony was out of my life, along with all his negative comments, I didn't feel like putting up with criticisms from anyone, especially Mom.

Once again resentments built and I hungered to let her have it, to tell her what a horrible mother she had been when I was little. Instead, I started counting the weeks until I would get away again. I ignored her as much as possible—which was impossible.

MY SECOND ESCAPE FROM MOM finally came in May after I completed all my junior college courses. This time I was moving to Lubbock where I would finish my degree.

On moving day I leaned into our red Mercury, buckled Alex and Andrea's seatbelts, started the car and pulled out, heading toward a new life, a huge grin plastered on my face. Each mile of scrub brush, cattle, cotton and oil fields I put between me and the gossips, the painful memories and Mom felt like a thousand pounds lifting from my shoulders. Halfway there, I started laughing. Soon we were all giggling as we started playing a game that had me honking at each tractor the kids spied and counted. Joy filled that car.

We settled into a small red brick rental house near the campus. After advertising for childcare help, I interviewed many ladies before settling on a sweet older woman who could pick up Andrea from nursery school and be there for Alex when he walked home from the nearby public school. Unbelievable. My imp was in the first grade.

THE FIRST THING I DID upon arriving on the flat, spread-out Tech campus was head to the Allied Arts Department to investigate how I could major in architecture. Harboring a long-time dream to one day design houses, I truly wanted to do this rather than teach school.

I entered the assistant dean's office with high hopes, sat down across the desk and poured out my dream of becoming an architect. He listened to my request, then in a condescending tone replied, "We have a very difficult five-year course of study. Only one-fourth of the male students who start in our architecture program graduate—and no woman ever has."

Those words hit my new no-man-is-going-to-control-me button. Frustration flared up and I started to retort: You just met the first one. Where do I sign up? But facing the reality of an extra year of school in the architectural program, followed by an apprenticeship, I realized I couldn't afford to challenge the good-ole-boy cartel. So I returned to the Applied Arts

School to focus on art education. In 1963 women who worked were expected to become teachers, nurses or secretaries.

The art curriculum included learning how to teach a variety of art mediums. I tackled my classes with gusto, from textile designing to throwing clay pots, to painting. My favorite became the lost-wax jewelry casting and metalsmithing classes, especially after discovering that pounding metal into artistic shapes is a good way to loosen long-harbored frustrations.

OUR VACATION AT THE END of that summer consisted of a week with my parents in the cool, pine forests in the mountains at Ruidoso, New Mexico. It turned out to be better than I expected. Mom didn't show any signs of being hyper for the six days we all shared a cabin. She played games with the children and managed to limit her corrections of me to only about two a day. The results: some fun memories of her and a pledge to myself to stop being as silently critical of Mom as she was audibly of me.

The children and I also traveled to spend some time with Gracie's family that now included a son and two daughters. Near in ages, the cousins had great times together— playing games, hide-and-seek or the guys making forts from which they would bombard the girls' fort. It was always lively around their house. Gracie and her husband had been very supportive of me throughout my separation and divorce, surprising me once with the gift of a much needed washer and dryer. I'm sure they could have used that money elsewhere, but nowhere was it more appreciated. Every time I loaded that washing machine I gave thanks for my thoughtful sister and brother-in-law. What a relief to stop dragging two children and bags of laundry to the laundromat.

AT THE END OF MY next semester at Tech, I taped ten drawings on the paneled dining room wall and stood back. Which five should I submit for my final life-drawing grade? I didn't notice Alex standing behind me scratching his chest.

"Mommy, I itch," he said.

"Uh-huh, I replied, taking two of the drawings down.

"Me too," piped up Andrea.

That's when I lifted one T-shirt, then the other. Red bumpy spots. Ugly blisters were starting to form on Alex's tummy. Chicken pox. Egad. What timing. Sick kids meant no school and no daycare—with my finals starting in only two days. Panic. My babysitter had a morning job and couldn't help me out. I didn't know anyone else in Lubbock to call. With trepidation I put out a distress call to Mom. Surprising me, she dropped everything and came and took care of them for several days while I finished art projects, papers and exams. Being able to count on her in this emergency caused me to reexamine my negative opinion of her. The fact that the kids seemed to enjoy her added another plus mark.

Later that year Mom returned to Lubbock to watch the children while I went to the state art education convention to try to secure an art teaching job. Interviewing with several school districts represented there, I received an offer to teach in a district near Dallas after graduation. Yes. A job. Teaching art. That put a bounce in my step—until I walked into my house.

Mom had rearranged everything. The dining table now occupied a different location; my sofa moved to a place I would never have put it. I really didn't mind that she had rearranged my furniture, I could put the items back, like Granny always did. However, a wave of irritation flowed over me when I opened a dresser drawer and noticed she had straightened and thus scrutinized everything in my personal drawers. I squelched the urge to say anything about it, and instead thanked her for being so helpful.

Before she left, Mom remarked, "Diane, you have to be a better housekeeper. The kids' closet was messy. And half of their clothes were in the hamper. And toys, scattered everywhere. How can you live like this?"

Anger flared and I replied with an edge in my voice, "I have to make choices, Mom. I'm working as hard as I can to be a good mom and a good student. Tell me, what do you think I should let slide when term papers are due and the laundry needs to be done? Which should I slack off on—my grades or laundry? Should I ignore the children's needs? Turn in my art projects late? Or should some of the housework just have to wait till later?" Mom looked stunned. Her eyes widened. She didn't reply, but her sigh and shake of the head told me I failed to live up to her expectations—again.

Wow, that was almost a confrontation. One would think that after standing up to Tony, doing so with Mom would have been easier. It wasn't. There were too many years of keeping silent, of knowing nothing I said would change her. Frustrated silence remained my default position.

Starting Over

Two months later, sitting on the sofa in my living room with the front door open, I heard a clank and a plop and spied the mailman leaving the front porch. Probably bills, I thought, closing my textbook and getting up to fetch them. I plucked several envelopes out of the metal mailbox on the wall and recognized Mom's handwriting on one. Turning it over, I slid my finger under the flap and pulled out several pages, expecting to read the latest local gossip. Her first sentence made me suck in my breath: You must have done something awful to make your husband leave you.

By the time I read three sentences I had to sit down. Surely she cannot mean this. I read the letter to the end. Read it again. Slumping down on my sofa, my thoughts darted and clashed, trying to fathom what I had done, or said, to set her off like this. Nothing.

Mom's words slanted up across the page, spilling into the margins. Three long pages detailed all of my shortcomings, especially my failed marriage. She elaborated on what a mess I had made of my life, how I had embarrassed them, how I was an expensive failure with two children and a costly education. She could certainly use that money for things she wanted to do. I obviously didn't try to make my marriage work. She was very, very disappointed in me. I had failed the family.

Her cruel, ugly letter blind-sided me, as unexpected as her slap years earlier. This slap hit my heart, stinging much worse than the one to my cheek.

I wondered: how can she be so vicious? She has to be having another spell. She is blunt to the point of being cruel and thinks whatever she says is right.

Acknowledging that Mom was having a spell didn't take the hurt out of her harsh words. Obviously she did not agree with the financial agreement Dad had made with me. Her own indiscriminate over-spending may have garnered a comment from Dad to slow her spending down—maybe that was the catalyst that had launched this missile.

I was doing the best I could, excelling in a state with low tuition and watching every dime. And I had made the Dean's List again. With my graduation occurring in January, I had been hired to become an Instructor and team-teach with the Dean during the spring semester—a definite honor. My paycheck would even cover our monthly expenses. What else did she expect me to do?

I put 'The Letter' in my desk drawer, but the words careened around in my head. Failed. Failure. Disappointment. Embarrassment. Although a hundred miles away, her voice of condemnation followed me as close as my shadow. My head hurt. My heart hurt more.

The next day I drafted, then rejected, retort after retort. Anguish isn't easy to express on paper. Sleep eluded me. Wrath overtook all other emotions, filling my thoughts with one imaginary explosive confrontation with her after another. Yet I knew confrontation never worked with her, especially when she was on those roller skates. In her hyper state, she knew the TRUTH and I needed to hear it. She always had her own cockamamie rationale as to why she made hurtful comments.

Two days later the solution as to how to respond to her popped into my head—I would mail her own letter back to her. Surely after reading it again and realizing how brutal, how vicious she had been, she would retract some of it. Or maybe even apologize.

Not a chance. When she opened the envelope and discovered her own letter, she told Dad I had just put the wrong letter in the envelope.

Dad read it. He called me the next morning from his office. He tried to soften my distress. We had a long talk about Mom. Her spells were getting worse. Still refusing to take any medication, she was becoming angrier and more contentious during them. Dad tried to console me, "I'll talk to her when she becomes more reasonable."

Again I pondered, what makes her this way? What causes these spells?

Months passed before I went back to visit them. The subject of The Letter never came up. It became one more silent barrier between me and my waning hope of ever gaining a positive comment from Mom.

IT MUST HAVE BEEN FATE that propelled me back home for another visit. What happened during that trip changed my life, my children's and their children's.

11

Epiphanies:
Changing Myself

T HE CHILDREN AND I WENT to North Creek for Thanksgiving. Staying in my childhood bedroom rather than the guest room, I decided to clean out the drawers. I started my archeological dig in the cupboard in the blue bathroom I once shared with Gracie. Opening a large black plastic trash bag I started tossing in crumbling corsages, high school football programs and even an ancient pair of hose that required—gasp—a garter belt. Pleased with my progress, I continued to scan and throw items out until I reached the bottom of the last drawer and picked up a yellowed piece of folded notebook paper.

Unfolding it, I noticed the cursive writing slanted in several wobbly directions, indicating the writer must be about second grade. Then the contents hit me, making me suck in my breath. It started: When I am a Mom I will not ... and contained a short list.

No. Not true. This can't be true. Oh God. What have I done to my children?

I was the seven year old. I wrote that list. And I was doing every awful thing on it.

My breath coming in gasps, I reread the list:

When I am a Mom I will not
   whip my children
   scream at them
   make them cry
   scare them
   tell them they do things all wrong

This hit me hard. I screamed at my children. Often. Way too often. I corrected their behavior many times a day with a loud angry voice. And I spanked them. Just last week I had lashed out and spanked both of them before finding out who really misbehaved. Of course I made them cry. And scared them.

My knees gave way. I dropped down hard on the blue padded stool, the paper shaking in my hand. I longed to deny the truth. How could I, of all people, not realize what I was doing? How could I act like her, knowing all too well the impact on a child?

Talk about a traumatic awakening, a stab in the heart. Going through the stress of a messy divorce, the pressure of school deadlines and single-parenting provided no excuses. My very own words reverberated back at me. This was one core-shaking jolt I would not, could not, ignore.

The primary difference between Mom's discipline and mine was that I spanked only with my hand, never a shoe or hair brush, never as hard as I could hit or more than three swats per spanking. That was no excuse either.

I stared in dismay at my stunned reflection in the vanity mirror, trying to rationalize that some of my behavior improved on hers. Yet in my heart I knew whose reflection stared back at me from that appalling mother-mirror.

I IMMEDIATELY STARTED TRYING TO change my behavior. Spankings stopped unless the child's actions were life-threatening, like the time four-year-old Andrea ran out into the street. My hardest habit to break was the tendency to yell at them. I became super-sensitive about how often I raised my voice. Way too often. As soon as I heard stridence in my voice I would stop, take a deep breath, sometimes several, before quietly resolving the situation. I broke up squabbling kids by sending them into different rooms before asking each, in turn, what happened. This gave all three of us time to cool hot tempers. My new calm soon gave Alex and Andrea confidence that their mother would listen to both of them before becoming judge and jury and dispensing any corrective action such as a time-out or putting away a favorite toy.

On the plus side, I instigated a special tuck-in routine of private time with each child before hugging and kissing them good-night. A special just-Mom-and-child moment.

Habits are hard to break. Research indicates it takes six weeks of a

Epiphanies: Changing Myself

repeated action to form a habit; it took much longer to break one. It turned out to be all too easy to backslide, to instantly raise my voice. It took months for me to halt my instant yelling. What a relief when I succeeded. Our lives changed. Much of the tension in our home diminished. The adrenalin rush and tension that hit my body when I got mad or yelled, dissipated. Single mothering became more of a joy, less of a stressful task.

How fortunate for my children that I wrote myself that list—and found it when I did. It broke the cycle of patterning my behavior after Mom's. That list to myself stopped her instant spankings and screaming from being passed on to the next generation. I have loved seeing my daughter Andrea, when her own young son misbehaved, getting down at his eye level and very quietly saying, "Josh, look at me," and then softly explaining to him what he needed to correct.

Now three generations have improved on the parenting skills of their own parents. Mom told me her parents had vicious, ugly, scary arguments, making her determined that her marriage would be different. No loud arguments. And she succeeded. My parents never exchanged heated words in my hearing. I, in turn, eliminated spankings, screaming and constant criticisms. Along with curtailing my negative parenting, I wish I had expanded my fledgling attempts to become a more affectionate parent. It also turns out to be hard to give what you didn't get—to imitate or initiate behavior you never received. My own children have bridged that emotional abyss. Along with quieter reprimands, they give my grandchildren many more supportive comments and compliments, plus a lot more hugs than they—or I—or Mom—received as a child.

As I tackled the challenges in my personal life, social and political challenges erupted throughout our country. The Sixties were violent. Blacks rose up against decades of oppression. Political conventions were surrounded by hostilities and chaos. Protestors against the Vietnam War started burning their draft cards and American flags and moving to Canada. Belligerent marches and riots occurred across the country.

Music changed from love ballads to lyrics like those in Bob Dylan's song about all the things that were a-changin.' As I embraced my single life in the midst of a country in turmoil, feminist stirrings around the country started a-changin' everybody's life. My awakened independence, my taking charge of my life, coincided with the beginning of the Women's Movement. Not only did I wake up, but so did my entire generation to the idea that we women should be treated as equals—equal humans, equal household responsibilities, equal parenting and equal pay for equal job opportunities—like becoming an architect.

Men balked. They liked their role as the head-of-the-house, like my ex-husband, a product of the Deep South where women were still expected to wait on and obey their husbands. I, of course, did not have to get any entrenched husband to change his ways.

I just needed to change myself.

TWO LIFE-CHANGING EPIPHANIES HIT ME like thunderbolts that year: the first, finding that childhood letter to myself; the second, the result of seeing a movie. Not long after that fateful visit home, I had a date with a new fellow to see the much talked-about movie *Dr. Zhivago.* I had no inkling that this Hollywood movie was about to change my life.

I sat in the darkened theater and watched Zhivago's tragic life unfold in glorious Technicolor with turbulent scenes of the Russian revolution that tore relationships and a country apart. Zhivago's foster family arranged for him to become a doctor and marry their daughter when what he really wanted to do, tried to do, was write poetry and live with Lara, his true love. On the way to see her, he was abducted and forced to participate as a doctor in the revolution. Afterwards, he tried, and failed, to find Lara. Throughout his life, time after time, year after year, Zhivago's attempts to exert any control over his life ended in futility.

My poor date—I barely spoke to him the rest of the evening. Struck by how much parents, culture, and political turmoil—like the revolution in Russia or the violent protests in our own country—could change the course of an individual's life, my mind churned with thoughts of what I did, and did not control in my life.

Arriving home, the date dismissed, the babysitter paid, the children asleep, I made myself a cup of tea and sat down on my sofa. With only the hallway light on, casting soft shadows around the living room, I scrutinized my life, trying to see clearly how family, fate and personal choices had affected the course of my life. My conclusion: since we cannot control others nor public

Epiphanies: Changing Myself 123

events that impact our lives, we should make every choice that we do control with great care. With this insight in mind, I evaluated my present and future. What or who influenced my decisions? What choices did I control?

First, I did not get to choose my mother, but I could choose to control my reaction to her and her constant criticisms. All I had to do to hear her critical voice was glance in a mirror. Even living two hours away from her, I would hear her lament, "Your hair. Do something with your hair." Or, "Change that top." Or, "Why can't you do anything right?"

I needed to learn how to listen to my own voice, not hers. From this moment forward, I vowed to ignore her hurtful words and actions that told me I was a failure, a disappointment, incompetent.

Second, I did choose my husband. I spent five woeful years married to him. Now, by dwelling on my hurt, resentment and anger at him, I had let caustic memories of our dysfunctional relationship affect two more years of my life—and he wasn't even in town. How stupid and unproductive.

Never again, I promised myself, would I let anyone destroy my self-esteem or hamper my personal goals. I was the one in charge of my life, my attitude, my appearance, my self-confidence and my emotions—not my ex-husband and not my mother.

Realizing how often my negative thoughts about Mom and Tony affected my happiness, I started trying to let go of painful memories. Each time a visual memory of a negative event with either of them popped into my head, I envisioned tearing that memory-photo into tiny pieces, flushing the fragments down the toilet, and watching them swirl out of my life. Each time a hint of their disapproving words started to replay in my mind, I visualized pulling the loops of tapes out of my mental tape recorder and throwing them on the floor of my carport. I saw myself bend over the tapes and strike a match. I watched as they shriveled and curled up as the flames devoured them, creating an acrid smell of fried, dead words. To complete their destruction, I mentally stomped on the charred pile. Fire out. Memory deleted.

I did a lot of mental flushing and stomping. Soon their negative images, and words came to mind less and less often. Never again would I dwell on the if-onlys or what might have been. The past was just that—the past that could not be changed. From this moment on, I would focus on the future, on my positive accomplishments and plans.

As months passed, this new direction held the promise of becoming even better. My goal of acquiring an education that would support my family would be completed soon. My bad mothering habits were changing. I began to feel good about myself, about my changes, my achievements. Finally a sense of warm contentment spread through me.

Mom didn't let it last.

My grand plan to let go of Mom's criticisms turned out to be much more frustrating and difficult to maintain than I expected. While Tony now lived in Georgia and contact between us rarely occurred, Mom's constant critique of me continued, spell or no spell. There were hundreds of comments, looks and frowns that needed to be flushed or burned, making it impossible to get rid of every one. Each new criticism knocked the scab off my old wounds, exposing me to the toxic enticement of anger, self-pity or revenge. Each trip home meant more criticisms. The struggle not to respond to her in a harsh way made me dread every visit, including one during the Christmas holidays.

With the car packed with suitcases and presents, the children and I headed to North Creek, playing our spy-the-tractors game during the drive. While driving I kept splaying my Sassy Pink fingernails out on the steering wheel, admiring my Christmas gift to myself—a rare, rare manicure. The manicurist suggested I try flat tips rather than rounded tips as this shape might stop my fragile nails from splitting into the quick so often. I had learned that my weak nails and thin hair, the cause of so many of Mom's negative comments, were due to my having a thyroid deficiency.

Reaching my parent's home, we filed into the house. Sniff. Yummm. Pot roast for dinner. Red candles and shiny gold ornaments on the dining table set the holiday mood, as did Bing Crosby crooning Christmas carols on the record player.

That night, while the five of us dined at the table in the den, Mom reached over and picked up my right hand. Scrutinizing my nails, she ran her finger along the flat tip. A disapproving frown settled on her brow. She put my hand back on the table with a sigh. The corners of her mouth turned down as she shook her head. I lowered my hands with their wrong-shaped nails into my lap, clenching them, and my teeth. A biting response leaped into my mind: I'm so glad my flat tipped nails have provided you with something new to criticize. Choking down this angry retort, I reminded myself: Let go Diane.

Epiphanies: Changing Myself

Let go. Her actions won't get to you unless you let them. Change the steps to this dance. Breathe. Let go.

I wanted to let go, to move out of Grudgeville, but after twenty-five years of reacting in silent anger to her hundreds of negative comments, shakes of her head, or disapproving looks, a lump of resentment, the size of Mount McKinley, had built up inside of me. I struggled to make my new resolve happen: to ignore her. I sat there wishing I could get up the nerve to say: Please Mom, approve of me, just once. Just one compliment. Why can't you do that? Would it be too hard to say just one positive thing? To maybe say that you like the color, even if you don't like the shape of my nails?

I didn't say it.

With a sudden insight I realized that Mom's inability to give me a compliment was truly sad. How sad that she had such a negative focus, always looking for something to criticize, to correct. But her critical mindset was her problem. It would not be mine anymore. Unclenching my hands, I took a deep breath, letting go, letting go, letting go.

RETURNING TO LUBBOCK, WE THREE heard January blow in that night, whistling and moaning as the wind whipped sleet and snow over the High Plains of the Texas panhandle. Squeals of excitement filled the house the next morning when the kids awoke and saw all that strange white stuff. Bundling up, we went out to make a snowman. It took all the snow in our small front yard to create one little two-foot-tall fellow. Still, with a red cowboy hat on his head and large navy buttons for his eyes, he looked fabulous to us.

The next day Alex started back to school and Andrea to daycare. I sat down at my desk, pulled open the bottom drawer and retrieved a folder labeled GRADUATE. Inside, well-worn, dog-eared sheets listed every class I had to take to achieve that goal. Every class, except four, had a big X crossed through it. Four more classes and I would be a college graduate. A contented feeling came over me as I recalled each completed step.

WHILE MY ACADEMIC LIFE TURNED out to be esteem-boosting, my dating life didn't. During my two years at Tech, hoping to have some fun, I started dating. While at first flattered when a man appeared interested in me, a single mother, I soon discovered why. I had several first-dates not to be followed by a second. It seems that even in this era when birth control and free sex became available, men still focused on divorcees as prime targets. Since I'd stopped dating at seventeen, my inexperience with sexually aggressive men landed me in several dicey situations. Horrified by their often blatant expectations, I let them know I wasn't fulfilling their fantasies.

Not wanting to get seriously involved with anyone, ever again, I fled any type of physical or emotional overture, especially from one fellow who made me think getting involved might be a good idea.

As graduation approached I had to choose whether to take that teaching position in the school district near Dallas or get a master's degree. With Dad's encouragement and support, I chose the latter for two reasons: my salary as a teacher would increase substantially and I would also be eligible to teach at the junior college level. With the encouragement and recommendation of a professor, I headed to California for a master's degree in art education.

California, here I come.

DAD HELPED ME DRIVE OUT to California that summer while the children went for their summer visit with their Georgia grandparents and father, now remarried—again.

The miles seemed endless, but blissfully silent. Both of us were enjoying being on a road trip together for the first time without Mom's ceaseless chatter. This would have been an opportune time to discuss Mom and her spells. We didn't. Dad never discussed how he coped with Mom's behavior during a spell with either Gracie or me. I do wish he had, but maybe he struggled with how to do so himself. No one knew, at that time, what caused her spells nor what to do about them.

During those hours I realized I had seldom been alone with my Dad. While he had not been one of those get-on-the-floor-and-play-with-the-kids type of dad, he had always been rock-steady, the kind of father you knew you could count on. Often absent, working long hours during my childhood, I did recall feeling safer when he was home. Although showy gestures of affection were not his style, with an occasional hug, Dad let me know he loved me. His actions—such as helping me drive all the way to California with a rental trailer swaying behind the car—secured that feeling. Having one parent I could count on made a huge difference in my life.

Epiphanies: Changing Myself   127

This move felt very different from the move to Lubbock. Then, with each mile, I felt lighter, free at last from the past, the bondage of my marriage and Mom. This trip, my spirits soared with excitement in anticipation of the future. I couldn't help but grin when I realized the distance between Texas and California meant no trips home for every holiday—and hopefully fewer calls from Mom. But as the wheels turned, anxieties about the challenges ahead kept revolving in my mind. Where would I live? Would Stanford be too hard? Would the children adjust?

As we rolled into Palo Alto, my anxiety reverted back to excitement. Of course the kids would adjust. Of course I would find a nice place to live. Of course Stanford would be too hard. But I could do it. I could do it all.

I hoped.

We went straight to the campus. At the sight of the sandstone buildings, arched walkways and red tile roofs, a huge grin planted itself on my face. I rubbed my arms to quell the goose bumps that popped up. At the bookstore I bought a local newspaper and searched the apartment ads looking for listings wanting a SWF roommate. A gut reaction of apprehension settled in my stomach as I jotted down a few phone numbers. Who would want a temporary roommate for only the weeks while my children were gone? What would the roommates be like? Younger? Smokers? Hippies? Slobs?

As we headed toward the student union, I spied a wooden kiosk full of flyers promoting everything from cars-for-sale to get-acquainted mixers. As I circled the round wooden structure, I spotted, almost hidden behind a flaming pink sheet advertising a Hare Krishna meeting, a white card: Wanted Female Roommate. Yes. I felt much more comfortable calling university coeds than strangers in the public newspaper—unless they turned out to be Krishnas.

The lively crowd of students crossing the Quad appeared to be a United Nations gathering of all races, sizes and ages. Males wearing flowing African robes and hippie-looking women in multicolored long skirts with flowers in their hair swished past me. This scene was so different from Tech where Caucasians, jeans and cowboy boots were the norm.

AFTER SIX THAT EVENING I called the apartment number.

"Hello," a pleasant voice answered. I explained my circumstances, including that I would be a temporary roommate. The female, named Ellen,

128   MOM, MANIA, AND ME

hesitated, then after a muffled conversation with her roommate, asked me to come over in about an hour. I jotted down the directions.

Dad went with me. We liked the looks of the complex that turned out to be only a mile from campus: dark redwood siding, balconies, nice landscaping, covered parking. We trudged up the stairs to the apartment on the second floor. A pretty blonde with a big smile answered our knock.

"Hello, welcome. I'm Ellen." Introductions to her roommate, an airline stewardess, followed.

I instantly liked them both. I just hoped they liked me too.

Ellen showed us through the immaculate apartment that had three bedrooms and a spacious living room with a balcony overlooking the huge pool in the courtyard. Dad and I settled down on the sofa for an exchange of backgrounds and situations. At the end of twenty minutes and twenty questions, she said, "Thank you so much for coming. We'll call you with our decision tomorrow evening as we have other candidates to consider."

Bummer. Going down the stairs, my spirits sank too. Where to look next? Then Dad, a keen observer of people and their reactions said, "They're going to accept you. They just need to confer to find out what the other thinks."

The next evening I stared at the phone, willing it to ring. Five-thirty. Six o'clock. I massaged my temples with my fingertips as I watched Walter Cronkite report the evening news. Checked my watch, again. Finally at 7:00 the phone rang.

"It's Ellen. We would like for you to move in. We hope you haven't found another place."

"No. Oh, I mean no, I haven't found another place. This is great. When may I move in?"

"Anytime."

By nine o'clock that evening, my new bedroom took on the look of a storage bin as Dad and I hauled up the score of boxes of personal and household items. My furniture remained back in Texas in storage. The next morning I hugged Dad goodbye before he got into a taxi to go to the airport. He seemed as pleased with my situation as did I.

I spent the rest of that day unpacking my personal items, setting aside my favorite blue sheath and matching blue flats to wear on my first day at Stanford.

Epiphanies: Changing Myself 129

The next morning, anticipation, excitement and adrenalin all surged though my body putting a bounce in my step as I walked up to the building to register for classes. What a different life this summer offered me—life as a single, unencumbered female sharing an apartment.

How different would it be? More than I ever imagined.

12

Good Things Happen

THE APARTMENT COMPLEX EMPTIED EARLY each day as the inhabitants, mostly single young professionals, headed out to work. Each afternoon I returned from classes to find a tempting swimming pool all to myself. After slipping into a swimsuit, I would head out to it, lugging textbooks to try to keep up with the momentous amount of reading required on the fast-paced quarter system. After slathering on lotion and plopping on my floppy red straw hat, I stretched out on a lounge chair, trying to soak up some sun and some knowledge. Later, feeling hot and sticky, I'd slip into that refreshing water, swim a couple of laps, then resume my bake-and-study position.

Each afternoon, another college student arrived poolside, interrupting my peace. An extra-tall guy, he currently attended a junior college after serving four years in the military. His conversations always started with the status of his application to transfer into the Stanford as a junior.

"I didn't hear again today," he grumbled.

"Sorry." I answered, marking my place on the page with my finger before looking up.

"Don't you think I should have heard by now?"

"I don't know," I replied daily. After a week of the same exchange, I asked, "Have you heard from any other colleges?"

"I didn't apply to any others," he said.

"Well good luck. Let me know when you hear." I said, returning to my reading. I thought: he's either very cocky or not very smart—or both.

After five o'clock, the deck chairs would begin to fill up with residents in swim attire. Beer and cards appeared, games started, shouts and sprays of water from water polo filled the air. Weekends found subgroups of us heading over the foothills to an old weather-beaten seafood restaurant on

Good Things Happen

the coast. There we feasted on fresh seafood, dripping with butter. Sometimes we strolled over to a nearby volleyball court for a raucous game.

What a contrast this lifestyle created for me, having spent evenings during my earlier college days playing games like Chutes and Ladders or Go Fish with two little people.

Many nights our apartment turned into the local gathering place after dinner. First one guy, then two or three females, then more fellows would wander in our open door, filling the seats and sprawling on the beige carpet. Our boisterous conversations wandered over a wide spectrum of topics. Would the Vietnam War ever end? President Johnson declared he wasn't running again? Who would? How could one part of the country be holding a massive love-in in Haight-Ashbury while violent race riots were erupting in Detroit, Atlanta and Cleveland? Was it really possible we could land a man on the moon?

Blond Eric, an engineer, usually turned up sometime during these evening before starting his job of tracking our new satellites across the late night sky. One night, he whipped out a new object to show us—a pocket sized calculator. The guys grabbed it and started examining the features. One, looked up and queried in awe, "How much does this cost?"

Eric grinned and boasted, "Well over a hundred dollars."

The technical revolution had started. The sixties and my life, while full of turmoil, were also filled with wonderful and exciting changes.

As much fun as this summer produced, my mommy genes missed those two kids. I eagerly awaited the end of my single days and the arrival of Alex and Andrea. Our family of three moved into campus housing—a two bedroom row house with durable vinyl furniture and gray tile floors—student housing sans frills. Each row of six units backed up to six more with a wide fenced courtyard between them providing a safe play area for the swarms of children living there. All Alex or Andrea had to do was walk out our back door and yell, "Anybody want to play?" Playmates would spill out of screened doors up and down the row.

One of the required courses for my degree started at three in the afternoon, the very time my children, now in first and third grades, came home from school. I was stymied as to who to hire and how to pay for a daytime babysitter for two hours every day for three months.

Rex, the tall Stanford applicant, stopped by our apartment often now that he had been accepted. After watching him patiently listening to Andrea's convoluted plans for a playhouse, an idea popped in my head.

"Rex, would you consider coming over at three every afternoon to watch the kids for two hours in exchange for dinner?"

We worked it out. He came and kept the bandages and Kool-Aid handy, often playing pick-up basketball games on a nearby court. Upon arriving home after class, I started dinner and we four ate together, becoming good friends over the dinner table. Sometimes he arrived carrying a roast for me to cook, an item beyond my budget. This arrangement worked out well for me, and the kids seemed to really like him.

After that term ended, Rex continued to stop by and we often took the kids to a park. While I found his wholesome all-American look, brown hair, hazel eyes and extra height of six feet five inches attractive, I viewed him as just a safe male friend since I was not about to get involved with a broke, younger, undergraduate student. Besides, I had begun casually dating several older graduate students. Rex, who had never been married, also considered me as a safe friend as he didn't want to get involved with an older divorcee with two children.

Mom seldom phoned, and as weeks passed with little contact I rarely thought about her. Angry memories popped into my consciousness less and less often. Then came this call: "I'm coming to see you."

My heart sank. I didn't have two extra seconds during the day with classes and papers exceeding my study time already. Somehow I managed to get the apartment extra clean, wondering why I bothered, expecting some stinging comments on my housekeeping abilities despite my efforts.

Mom arrived and surprised me. Her three-day visit actually turned out to be rather pleasant. The children were a delightful age: Alex nine, Andrea six. Mom played board games with them while I studied. On Saturday we took her sightseeing in San Francisco. On the fishy smelling wharf, Andrea all of a sudden exclaimed, "I smell chocolate." Our noses followed the tantalizing smell, ending up at the Ghirardelli Chocolate Factory—a yummy hit with all of us.

That evening, while finishing the dishes in the kitchen, I heard a knock on the screen door, followed by a familiar voice— Rex's. I introduced him to

Good Things Happen

Mom, explaining his role as my babysitter. She did a real double-take. After he left, she turned to me, "He seems nice but I've never heard of such—having a man for a babysitter."

"Yes," I replied, "I guess it is unusual, but it has worked out for us."

She shrugged but didn't shake her head or put on that disapproving look she had perfected. Rex had obviously made a good impression.

On this trip, Mom only made a few mild criticisms of me, the children and the apartment. I considered that maybe, maybe, she was starting to change or at least stop mothering-correcting me constantly. Maybe, maybe, she viewed me as an adult now and we would have a better relationship in the future.

I hoped so.

ONE EVENING, SEVERAL WEEKS LATER, Rex shocked me by asking, "Why don't you stop seeing other guys?"

Startled, I retorted, "Why would I do that? You don't take me out."

His request puzzled me. We were in no way romantically connected. We didn't date as he was too broke for dates—and picnics in the park with the children didn't count as a date in my mind.

Several weeks after Rex's request, an attorney invited me to go up to San Francisco to see a stage production—on a real date. As I sat there in the dark, enthralled by the performance, I thought, I can't wait to tell Rex about this. Rex. I wanted Rex to share this event with me, not the rich, handsome lawyer by my side. What was I thinking? What did this feeling for Rex mean? Stunned, feelings in a turmoil, alarmed that I might be falling in love with Rex, the rest of the performance ended in a blur.

After tucking the kids in bed the next evening, I asked Rex, "What did you mean when you asked me to stop seeing other fellows?"

"Nothing, don't worry about it. Go ahead. Go out with them."

And thus started our see-saw romance. One minute I wanted to focus only on Rex, the next, I felt too scared to even contemplate it. When I warmed to the relationship, he cooled off. When he turned warm, I turned cool.

We were both surprised at the change of emotions over the next year. I, who vowed never to marry again, began cautiously to love again. The protective igloo stacked around my heart started to melt, only to re-freeze, but each time I warmed up, the igloo became smaller. Still, I kept wondering, can I trust any man with my love? As the months went by, my answer turned from doubt to confidence, that yes, I could trust and love Rex.

By the time he reached the middle of his senior year, I had completed my degree. Not wanting to rush into a commitment, but not ready to end our relationship, I took an art teaching position in nearby San Jose rather than returning to Dallas. Finally, that November, we both warmed up at the same time. Rex proposed, and without any reservations, I said, "Yes."

That Christmas holiday, Rex, my two children and I drove non-stop from California to Texas. I silently figured that if our relationship could withstand the challenges of a long car trip with two feisty kids, we had a chance to make a marriage work.

With my entire family gathered in the jungle room, Rex and I announced, "We're engaged." Gracie jumped up and hugged me. Grins and cheers came from everyone. After six single years, Diane had finally found a man.

"When are you getting married? Where will the wedding be?" Mom asked.

"In May, after Rex graduates," I said. "We haven't made specific plans yet."

At that statement, Mom went into take-over mode. Plans bubbled out of her mouth. "How about here? I could . . . blah, blah, blah." I tuned her out, immediately convinced we needed to keep control of our own wedding. Thus, a week later, back in Palo Alto, we called our families one morning to tell them we were getting married that afternoon, assuring them that they were still welcome to come in May.

HAVING EXPERIENCED THE DEVASTATION OF feeling unloved and unlovable since hiding in fear from Mom in my childhood, plus the rejection of my ex-husband, I relished the difference when Rex hugged me. His hugs worked like an etch-a-sketch eraser, instantly wiping out all those unlovable feelings. To this day, when he pulls me toward him until my head rests on his shoulder and his arms envelop me tenderly, a surge of affection engulfs my entire being. How safe I feel. How protected. How wanted, needed, loved, cherished. At last I know what being loved—and loving back—feels like.

While our marriage has not been without challenges and hurdles over the years, being the object of Rex's affection remains a constant. As our years together lengthen, our romance continues to be tender and loving. We make sure to give each other a special hug every day—a simple expression of our feelings for each other. Those hugs feel delicious, like biting into a warm brownie fresh from the oven—and every day at our house is brownie day.

Marrying Rex came with a bonus—I gained a wonderful mother-in-law. Carrie, who could make any piano rock, loved to laugh and make others feel loved and appreciated. Our first encounter turned out to be a bit stand-offish, but I couldn't blame her. I'm sure no mother wishes her son would grow up and marry a ready-made family. But once the "I do's" were uttered, she welcomed me warmly, thus starting a loving relationship that I came to treasure. What fun to call her up and laugh together over something, anything that had occurred.

Why couldn't my relationship with Mom be more loving? Why couldn't we share hugs and laughter? While many of the fractures in my heart began to heal, I still longed for the hole in my heart named Mom, the deep one, to be filled with loving words and gestures from her.

ELEVEN FAMILY MEMBERS DID TAKE us up on the invitation to come and visit that May. They all came within seven days of our move to Washington, D.C. where Rex had a government job for the summer. Teaching art in a junior high in San Jose until Friday of that week, I wondered how we could possibly be ready to move that Saturday. Thus, in preparation for the company and the move, Rex and I packed and stacked about twenty boxes against the stairway wall before our guests arrived.

Ring. Ring. Knock, Knock. Knock. Alex and Andrea ran to the door, opening it to reveal Mom and Dad. A waft of White Shoulders fragrance proceeded Mom into the living room. In the midst of greetings Mom spied our wall of boxes. She stopped talking in mid-sentence, "What's all this?"

"The moving van comes this Saturday morning. We wanted to have time to have fun while you were here, so we packed some things early," I said.

Mom didn't understand why I had to do that. Every time she walked past them, I saw her disapproving look and shake of her head. I knew what she was thinking: how I could possibly entertain guests with ugly moving boxes stacked like that in my living room?

This was Rex's first visit from my parents after our marriage. He knew all about Mom's disapproving and take-charge nature; thus, it was fascinating to watch the first struggle of wills erupting between them. The issue: who would take Andrea to buy new shoes.

Mom motioned to Dad, "Come on, Edward," she said, pulling on her bright coral-colored coat, "We're going to take Andrea to get some new shoes."

Rex, rising, said, "I'm taking her, Mrs. Dweller."

"Oh, no, I'm going to take her," Mom stated. She beckoned to Andrea who looked confused as she glanced back and forth between them. So did I. So did Dad.

"Come on Andrea," Mom said.

Towering over his mother-in-law, Rex paused, then in a don't-challenge-me voice declared, "No, Mrs. Dweller, you're not. I'm taking her."

Mom's eyes grew big. She stood there staring at Rex who stared back. She finally broke eye contact. Dad's eyes widened. We had all become accustomed to giving in to her. If Dixie wanted to do something, she always got her way. None of us ever said "NO" to her. I couldn't keep from grinning as I watched her reaction when Rex said, "NO."

Mom never again challenged Rex.

WHAT A FUN BUT HECTIC week we had with Rex's parents, sister and husband, my parents, Gracie, her husband and their three children all coming and going at different times. That Friday, I survived the last day of teaching art in that challenging ghetto school. I watched the clock, eager to get home to finish packing the last boxes. Lists of lists were double checked as some items were going to storage in Michigan, our next home, some boxes were going with us to Washington, D. C. and some stuffed suitcases went to Georgia with the children.

Early Saturday, after the children left for their weeks with their Dad and the movers loaded the truck, we weary newlyweds started the long drive to Washington. Rex had taken a civil service exam earlier that spring, and after a flurry of telegrams from the White House had been selected to participate in a special government internship during the summer.

What a turn my life had taken. I never expected to fall in love again, much less marry my children's babysitter or live in Washington D.C.

What an incredible summer. Rex attended weekly meetings with various cabinet secretaries. On a daily basis he worked on special projects at the

Good Things Happen

Defense Department. We even had dinner at the White House. At the end of that summer we headed to Michigan where Rex started his advanced degrees while I taught art in the public schools in a nearby town. Alex and Andrea became active in school, sports and social activities. Days and months flew by. We were all very busy.

AFTER REX AND I MARRIED I made him a gold wedding ring. I formed the wax model, cast it at my dentist's office and buffed it up with a hand drill. That is when I had the bright idea that I would put him through graduate school making wedding rings. In Michigan, after purchasing the basic equipment needed to start my wedding ring business, I placed an ad in the student newspaper for custom designed wedding rings. Wow. The response all but overwhelmed me. After teaching art all day in the public schools, cooking dinner and tucking the kids in bed at each night, I went to work in my closet-studio. Over the next six years I learned about the challenges of running a business, including what the term "overhead" meant. It meant I didn't earn very much. But I loved every creative minute, especially watching the faces of beaming couples as they tried on their wedding rings for the first time.

DURING THE YEARS WE CALLED Michigan home, I didn't pay much attention to Mom's life, nor wonder how she was doing. Her weekly letter reported she stayed busy serving on the Salvation Army Board and volunteering at the Rehab Center and on the church visitation committee. During normal times, she was a wonderful worker, contributing time, effort and money to numerous community projects. Early in a spell she could be very productive.

Gracie clued me in on what happened during one of Mom's take-charge times. As Chairman of the local Litterbug Campaign, Mom decided something should be done about the creek north of town, long neglected and trashed. Mom organized the city maintenance staff, a concrete company, the Boy and Girl Scout Troops, the Garden Clubs and numerous good citizens, plus Gracie's family, and in one day the creek was transformed. All the litter disappeared, replaced with walks, benches, flower beds and shaded picnic areas. When Dixie became hyper-focused on a task, it got done, and done well.

DURING THE STRESSFUL PARTS OF Mom's spells that continued to occur, Dad coped with her without complaint. I was out of her life; she out of mine—except for short visits each year. Fortunately most of our time together lasted only about five days and occurred between her spells. Brushing off her negative comments became easier, but no more pleasant. Hearing Rex's counterpoints helped.

Mom: "You did that all wrong."

Rex: "Thank you for doing that."

Mom: "Your hair . . . Your outfit . . . Your . . ."

Rex: "You're beautiful."

Mom: giving me her disgusted look, shaking her head, indicating I disappointed her again.

Rex's face lighting up at the sight of me.

THE GRANDCHILDREN'S OPINION OF THEIR grandmother differed from mine and Gracie's. They considered their Grandmother Dweller great fun. Once when Gracie and I were both in town, we left Mom watching our five school-aged children while we went to retrieve her banged-up Buick from the body shop. Upon returning to the house thirty minutes later, we were perplexed to discover that Mom and all five grandchildren had disappeared. Where could they be? We searched the house looking for a note. None found. We hiked around the hillside and checked out the sandstone formation. No children anywhere. Stumped as to where they had vanished, we finally started calling some neighbors and then friends. An hour later they finally appeared—riding a Shetland pony. Mom had asked a farmer to bring it to her house. The kids had been having a blast taking turns riding it the ten blocks to the drugstore to get ice cream cones.

One spring while we lived in Ann Arbor my parents flew to Cleveland for a medical meeting. I drove down to see them. Mom waved to me as I came through the lobby door. Grabbing me by the arm she said, "Hurry up, we have to catch the commuter train."

I handed the bellman my bag. "Hold that for me," I yelled at him, hustling, trying to keep up with Mom's rapid walk for the next three blocks. Jabbering over her shoulder about an omelet she ate for breakfast that tasted unbeliev-ably yummy, she whisked me onto the metro.

"What are we doing? Where are we going?" I asked as we found seats.

"To the Cleveland Clinic,"

"Why are we going to the Cleveland Clinic?"

"Oh Diane, I remember they have the most inspiring angels going up the wall of their chapel and I want to make a pattern of them to take back to our church to put up in the foyer to the sanctuary," she said, waving her hands up in the air like an ascending angel.

With a sinking heart I realized her rip-roaring excitement probably indicated a spell.

Arriving at the clinic, Mom hustled to the front desk, "May I speak to the clinic manager please?"

"May I ask the purpose?" the receptionist asked.

"I need his help with a project for my church," Mom said. This garnered a puzzled double-blink from the lady.

"Please wait over there. I'll see if he is available." Mom and I took the two remaining chairs around a low glass coffee table.

Mom's animated speech and hand gestures continued. I noticed other people sitting nearby sneaking glances at her as she launched into this story in a spirited voice that carried well beyond our seating area.

"I went over to Mildred's, and the cutest young man brought something to her. He was so handsome. Dark hair and eyes. Just adorable. Anyway he came roaring up on a motorcycle. I'd never ridden on a motorcycle and I thought, 'Why not?' So I asked him to take me for a ride. I climbed on behind him, and off we went." A mischievous grin flashed across her face as she added, "I had to hold onto him around his waist."

"Where did you go?" I asked, not sure I really wanted the details.

"We went all the way around Lookout Mountain. You should have seen my hair when we returned," she confided with a loud laugh, sweeping her hands through her tightly permed, still-dark hair.

My mind envisioned that scene. Without a doubt, she had loved every second of it.

THE CLINIC MANAGER APPEARED, WELCOMING us into his office with a smile and handshake. His face developed a somewhat wary look by the time Mom finished explaining her goal with enthusiastic gusto. He did prove to be a terrific sport though, asking his staff to fetch us a tall ladder and some art supplies to accomplish the task. I went along with it. Teetering high up on the ladder, trying to reach and trace the outlines of the soaring angels without falling, I glanced down, catching the glances and raised eyebrows of the manager and staff behind Mom's back. Over the years I had seen many a puzzled look as people stared after her as she swept by them, intent on accomplishing one of her zany ideas. It made me sad to see her like this and know what others were probably thinking.

Early the next morning, Dad hugged me goodbye and left for his meetings. Later, as Mom and I stood at the curb next to my car, the familiar parting scene, repeated every visit, played out. We smiled at each other, said nice things like "Good to see you again. Enjoyed our visit . . ." There were no goodbye hugs. Only a wave of our hands, and off I went.

As I slid behind the steering wheel a painful knot settled between my shoulder blades. The impact of being in the presence of this galactic force-field, high-strung-motor-mouth almost rendered me unable to drive. Leaving her presence felt like I had switched off the vibrations of a boom box playing at Mach volume for the past twenty-four hours. Slowly, mile after mile, the total silence marred only by the sound of swishing tires on the highway, my tension began to loosen.

Watching my dad's calm demeanor in dealing with her during our visit, I concluded he had to be a saint. How did he stand to stay with her?

I noticed on my next visit to her church there weren't any angels watching over us. I never asked her what happened to that idea. Like so many, it evaporated when she calmed down.

Again I wondered: What goes through her mind when she has a spell? What causes them? Why does she get so wound up? Why? Will we ever have an answer?

My relationship with Mom grew more placid as we weren't often together, nor did she call often due to her dislike of paying "those ridiculous long distance charges." I maintained my goal of minimizing any prolonged interaction with her. I simply ignored Mom—until something weird happened to me, catapulting the need to understand what caused her spells to the top of my list.

13

Chemical Turmoil

REX LEANED OVER TO GIVE me a kiss, tears welling in his eyes, the lusty cry of our newborn daughter ringing in our ears. After four long years of disappointments, we were thrilled to finally welcome Shannon, a beautiful, healthy baby girl into our family.

Six months after her birth, I went to see the new young internist who replaced my retired doctor. After reviewing my records, he announced, "I doubt you need to take this thyroid supplement. It became almost a fad in years past to put women on thyroid pills."

"Are you sure? I've been taking it since I was diagnosed at age ten. My father, a doctor, tested me regularly."

"Well there is one way to find out. We'll pretest you now, then decrease the amount of thyroid you take over several months until you are off of it. Then a post-test will confirm how active your own thyroid gland is."

Against my gut reaction, I agreed.

Big mistake. Enormous mistake.

By the end of the fourth month of decreasing my dose of thyroid supplement, I sat on the edge of my bed begging my tired legs, tired arms, tired lungs and tired thoughts to perk up. An alarming amount of hair covered my pillow case and clogged the shower drain. My hands and feet were so cold I loved getting into a car that had been parked in the sun for hours, to feel the warmth start to flow into my icy fingertips in that auto-oven. Barely able to drag myself around to take care of the baby, I had to let Alex and Andrea, now teenagers, often fend for themselves.

At the end of the thyroid withdrawal period, the repeated blood test confirmed I was a classic example of hypothyroidism—a condition in which my defective thyroid gland caused bodily functions to teeter on the edge of dysfunction. I needed that thyroid supplement—and always would. But instead of giving me my former pill, made from a dehydrated cow's thyroid gland, this doctor decided to replace it with a new synthetic, but more stable thyroid pill—at the same dosage.

Gigantic mistake. Colossal mistake.

The third month on the new thyroid prescription I suspected I might be pregnant. All the early symptoms were there—two weeks late for my period, emotionally fragile and with very tender breasts. I went to see my gynecologist. Nope. No baby. The next month, once again pregnancy symptoms emerged. Again, no pregnancy. Then my behavior really started to change. Instead of two or three days of premenstrual syndrome (PMS) symptoms each month, now, for two horrible weeks prior to my period I turned into the Wicked Witch of the West. Dark circles surrounded my eyes making me look like Alice Cooper. If I wasn't screaming at everyone, I was crying about every little thing. I became aggressive, angry, irritable, anxious and just plain mean.

Having PMS for a couple of days prior to each period, my family and I could survive. But *two* weeks of severe PMS every month? I kept exploding like a PMS time bomb.

After my period would start, Glinda the Good Witch appeared, loving everyone and all of life—happy, cheerful, caring. Two weeks later during my ovulation time, the circles would reappear and my fangs emerge. I felt utterly powerless to control my emotions. I became frightened. Bewildered. This vicious cycle had to stop. I called and made an appointment with the internist and had to wait two weeks—two long, screaming, threatening, crying weeks.

Arriving at the doctor's office, I took a seat on a green vinyl chair and picked up a tattered magazine, something about golf. The words blurred as I struggled to hold back the tears. Minutes dragged by. Half an hour, then an hour. All my tissues were soggy. As soon as I entered the examination room the dam burst and I dissolved into body shaking sobs. Between gasps for air I tried to explain the hell I was living, trapped in. "It has to be the thyroid pill you put me on as nothing else has changed."

"I doubt the new pill has anything to do with your behavior," he stated emphatically, "but I'll order another thyroid test."

All the thyroid tests came back normal.

But I wasn't.

My children started disappearing from my presence, like I used to disappear from Mom's. I apologized, promising them and myself every month that I would be nicer. Month after month, I failed miserably. Rex took the brunt of my anger, confused as to who this banshee was.

I hated the feeling that I was out of control, taken over by someone else I didn't recognize and abhorred. For two weeks each month I felt like the ghoulish lost soul screaming in Edvard Munch's painting. I started to wonder if I might be possessed by a demon like those people in the Bible.

This is what my daughter Andrea recalls about my behavior during these months.

The first incident:
When I was about 13 or 14, I think it was around dinner time, you got frustrated about something, or had an argument with Rex—I really don't remember what started it, but you really flew off the handle, very uncharacteristic of you. You were in the kitchen and from the table I could see your face all contorted with anger and you were shouting something about how you couldn't take this anymore, you hated this (whatever this was). You screamed, "I'm leaving," and grabbed your keys, purse and coat and left. I felt very concerned and a bit unnerved about this—Shannon was in her high chair, and I remember looking at her and figuring I guess I'll take care of her tonight. Later when I asked you where you went you said you went to a drive-in and watched a double feature.

The second incident:
I came in from being out with a friend and as I got to my room I could hear you through your bedroom door crying. You were absolutely sobbing, like something horrific had happened. I didn't know what to do, but your door was closed so I left you alone.

Both incidents were atypical of your behavior.

144   MOM, MANIA, AND ME

MY TURBULENT BEHAVIOR CONTINUED. BACK to the doctor I went. Sitting there on the cold examining table in a flimsy cotton examining robe, again sobbing uncontrollably, I implored him, begged him, "Please find out what is wrong. I cannot keep living on this mad roller coaster, nor can my marriage survive it."

He tested my thyroid again and once more reported everything was normal.

Normal? Yeah, for Hell. I felt trapped in a netherworld I could not control, could not escape. A sneaky thought of suicide scared me. How can I survive thirty or forty more years of this? I have to get better. I can do it if I try harder. I can't stay stuck in this up and down cycle. I'm getting like Mom. Oh God. Please not like Mom.

I held onto what sanity I could, trying to behave better, failing each month. I hated myself. I knew I acted terrible. I struggled to curtail my ugly behavior, my ugly words.

Would I ever be normal again? How? When?

Several months later, during this state of physical and emotional turmoil, we added more stress to the situation by moving. Fortunately it was to beautiful Vancouver, Canada, for Rex's first job as a professor at the University of British Columbia. Our new home, perched on a hillside in West Vancouver, gave us a panoramic view of the city, the shipping channel leading to the docks in Vancouver—and the beach.

After the rental trucks were emptied and returned, I couldn't wait to get Shannon, now three, and me, down to that beach. Finally finding the box marked "Bathrooms," I grabbed two towels plus a spoon and plastic cups for Shannon to play with in the sand. We climbed in the car and headed down the steep street to the seaside. As we descended to the lower level, I sniffed, and sniffed again. The unique scent of the cedar trees that surrounded our house had been replaced by the briny smell of saltwater and sea life.

The beach was wonderful—sandy, white, uncluttered. Seagulls soared overhead. Their cries created a melodious backdrop to the chatter and delightful squeal of my toddler every time the foaming waves tickled her toes. Finally, a day of smiles.

STILL EXPERIENCING MY FORTNIGHTLY ANGST, as soon as the kitchen items were unpacked and the fridge stocked, I made an appointment with a local doctor. I hoped he would put me back on my old thyroid pill.

The Canadian doctor listened to my still tearful tale of woe, tested my thyroid again, perhaps with a different blood test and immediately determined that the dosage of the new thyroid medication was wrong. He reduced it to one-fourth of the amount I took—and an unquestionable miracle occurred in the next few months. Life became not only bearable again, but incredibly wonderful with exciting surprises. My hands and feet felt warm for the first time in my entire life. My quirky periods became regular. The inner turmoil vanished. The roller coaster came to a stop. I learned to laugh again.

What a difference the wrong and right amounts of one tiny pill had made in all our lives.

My seismic upheavals had been caused by taking too much of a medication to replace a missing natural body chemical.

Did my changed thinking and feelings duplicate in any way Mom's changes during her spells? She also took a thyroid supplement. It appeared she could no more stop her periodic ascensions to Planet La La than I could stop turning into that dreaded Thyroid-a-saurus every month.

What could be stimulating her behavior, causing her body and brain to act like it does? Could there be a pill she needs? Or one she should stop? During a spell did Mom feel like I did? Out of control? Helpless to stop the changes? Did she even realize her personality and behavior changed?

I had never before considered how Mom might view her spells. For the first time I considered her inability to control her behavior with some understanding. A hint of compassion found a small place in my heart.

I shared my experience and questions with Dad. He did extensive medical research to no avail. Mom's behavior was not linked to any pill she was taking, and in the early 1970s no medications were available in the United States for symptoms like hers other than drugs like the zombie-making Thorazine she now adamantly refused to take.

Mom's episodic eccentric spells and behavior continued.

"Diane, I just bought a house," Mom exclaimed in an exuberant voice. Her long distance call during peak phone rates instantly clued me in as to which planet she was on. "I was driving in the Highland area and they were having an open house, so I went in. It's exactly what we need and it's so cute

I bought it. Our house is too big for just the two of us. I love it. It's darling. Can't wait to show it to your dad."

A heavy sigh escaped from my lips. She had bought a house without even showing it to Dad, in less time than it took her to buy a pair of shoes. While it cost some money, Dad finally got the contract nullified. Her spells were definitely getting worse each year.

How much worse?

We were about to find out.

When I called home one evening to discuss the details of my upcoming visit, Mom sounded peculiar—dull, barely responding in quiet whispers—totally un-Dixie-like. When I arrived, the sight of her stunned me. An alien had taken over my peppy sixty-three-year-old Mom. She sat unmoving, expressionless in her chair at the breakfast room table, her still-dark hair looked unkempt, uncurled, unbrushed. Food dribbles stained the front of her blouse. She didn't have any lipstick on.

I sat down across from her. "Hello Mom."

She wouldn't at look me.

"Mom, how are you feeling?" No response.

"Mom?" My throat contracted. Who was this stranger?

"MOM?" Her eyes glanced toward me, then away.

"Is there something I can get for you? How about a coke?" I asked.

No answer.

"Do you want a coke?" Finally a negative shake of her head.

What had happened to her pride in her appearance? Her constant chatter? She took several moments to answer even the simplest questions. None of us had ever seen her act like this. She was in a profound, acute depression.

Prior to this deep depression, normal actions had been her version of a depression, especially when compared to her super hyped-up behavior during her spells.

Dad took her to Dallas to a psychiatrist. Months passed before the mother and the exuberant spells we all recognized returned.

This was the first and only depression Mom ever experienced in the ninety-two years she lived. This was the "little depression" she described to Dr. Fisher during our visit to the State Mental Hospital in 1976, just after Dad died, prior to my return to Canada.

14

Diagnosis
and Hallelujahs

I BOARDED THE PLANE IN DALLAS for my flight to Canada at the end of the month I stayed in North Creek to help Mom after Dad's funeral. Plopping my weary body into my seat, I collapsed with total physical and emotional exhaustion. It wasn't long until the monotonous drone of the engines lulled me to sleep. But snatches of the past month kept surfacing in my subconscious—leaving the cemetery in a hurry ... Mom wanting to buy an airplane ... moving the trust to another bank ... calling Dr. Fisher ...

A child giggled behind me. A different giggle chimed in. Sitting up, blinking, I looked out at the puffy clouds covering the horizon below the plane. An attendant smiled as she walked down the aisle, checking that seatbelts were fastened for our landing in Vancouver.

At least my flight had been smooth, much smoother than my mind. I still could not grasp the fact that Dad had died.

Grief, held in check during this last month surged up, overwhelming, threatening to reduce me to a blubbering lump. Tears spilled over the rims of my eyes. Sucking in a deep breath, pressing a tissue to my eyelids, I tucked the pain down deep—again. I'd deal with it later. Soon. But as my plane touched down all I could think about was how much we were going to miss him. And worry about how Gracie and I were going to contain Mom's behavior during her spells. Leaving her in the midst of this spell had my stomach in knots. What shenanigans will she pull without the Dad-brake to keep her in check?

What Mom did shocked me.

One evening, a week after returning home, Rex hollered upstairs, "It's your mom on the phone."

Oh Lordy. Is she okay? Picking up the kitchen phone, I chimed, "Hi Mom. How are you?"

"I'm doing fine."

"What are you doing?" I asked with trepidation.

"Well, Dr. Fisher called and I went back to see him. He prescribed a new pill that has recently become available.

What's it for?"

"It'll keep me from going into a depression," she said. "Can't say I can tell any difference yet, but then I don't feel depressed. This is in case I might have one."

"What's it called?

"Lithium."

"Mom, I'm so glad he called and he's helping you. He seemed so nice." Crossing my fingers, I asked, "Will you keep seeing him?"

"Well, I'll have to go back every so often and get a blood test about this pill."

Hanging up the receiver later, I stood there a second before shouting, "Hallelujah" and breaking into a happy dance around the dining table. "Mom's seeing the psychiatrist. She's got pills, she's got pills," I chanted, giddy with hope. My family looked at me like I'd lost my mind.

Maybe, just maybe this will help with her spells. At least now I don't feel so guilty about tattling on her to Dr. Fisher.

But what is lithium? When I left Mom a week ago, the new widow definitely did not act depressed. Why give it to her if she isn't depressed? Wanting to understand the what-and-why of it, I went in search of information at the University of British Columbia Medical School.

Driving across Lions Gate Bridge, I followed the circuitous street through the towering cedar trees in Stanley Park. Swinging west via many turns on crowded streets I finally reached the university medical library. There, articles in the latest medical journals offered some clues.

Struggling through the medical lingo, I read that the nerve endings in our brains connect thoughts using electrical charges called synapses. Without the right balance of chemicals, like lithium salts, the chemistry of the brain changes, triggering strange connections that result in eccentric behavior, like Mom's.

Diagnosis and Hallelujahs 149

The use of lithium had recently been approved in the United States to treat people with something called manic-depression, a mood disorder. Lithium salts helped to balance the chemistry in the brain, stabilizing mood swings in both directions—it would keep people from getting too manic or too depressed.

Fabulous news. Mom's body evidently does not maintain the correct chemical balance in her brain. A small pill of lithium salts, a basic element, taken every day, is all she will need to stabilize her erratic brain chemistry and subdue her manic moods.

It was a relief to understand that her spells and hyper behavior were due to chemistry that would now stay in balance. And I understood firsthand how critical it was to get body chemicals that got out of whack, back in balance.

With lithium, Mom's brain chemistry could become stable.

A shaft of sunlight hit the long library table where I sat fantasizing about what life without Mom's spells would be like. No more wild spending sprees. No more wrecks. No more wearing us down with pie-in-the-sky plans and jabber. A tiny pill of hope called lithium had just brightened our family. It would change all of our lives, not just Mom's. The weight of the despair of not knowing what to do about her spells lifted from my shoulders. A grin swept over my face until a feeling of sadness seeped into my excitement. Why couldn't this have happened while Dad was alive? Why didn't he get to enjoy life with Mom without all the frantic activities like the house buying episode?

I CALLED GRACIE AS SOON as I got home.

"Gracie, Mom went back to see that psychiatrist I told you about. He's given her a pill called lithium that will keep her from getting depressed. And— you better sit down—it will keep her from getting hyper too. No more spells. Can you imagine Mom acting normal all the time?"

Phone silence lasted a moment before she replied, "No, I can't. Are you sure it will work?"

"The literature states it will as long as she takes it."

"You know how she hates pills. What happens if she stops it?" she queried.

"I don't know. Let's hope we never find out."

The relief that flooded through the whole family was like Noah seeing a rainbow after a storm that lasted forty years, not just forty days. Our constant fears of a crisis neither she, nor we, could control, was gone. At last she will be normal.

If she takes that pill.

It worked. Mom appeared to be stable throughout the next year. No hyper spells the doctor referred to as manic episodes were evident. She still criticized me, but her ability to sleep, to speak calmly, and to shop and drive responsibly were all improved by that little pill. Side effects that could include a change in heartbeat, stiffness, tiredness, headache, nausea, tremor, weight gain, dizziness or seizures were not evident, but she did complain of being thirsty often. After the drugged effect of Thorazine, a little thirst was acceptable.

"WHAT CAN I DO?" BECAME Mom's frequent question during the year after Dad's funeral. She wanted to do something useful, something that would benefit others. "I can sit around a bridge table when I get old," my sixty-six year old mother declared.

Mom decided to update her nursing credentials. She had to arrange to get a special dispensation, due to her age, to attend classes. It helped that she knew the head of the hospital that offered the training. Off she went to stay in a dorm (keeping the lights on all night), attending classes and wearing a crisp white nurse's uniform again. She even donned the starched white cap with the black band on it, designating her status as a Registered Nurse. The change in the younger nurses' uniforms to colorful, printed, hospital attire exasperated her. "I don't understand why they don't wear white uniforms and their nursing caps. They are certainly not professional looking," became her repeated criticism.

I could tell by the lilt in Mom's voice that she loved her training, including how to use a blood pressure cuff, an invention introduced in the forty years she had been away from nursing. "Pharmaceuticals have changed greatly, "she said, "but sick people need exactly what they needed when I trained—someone to help them feel better."

Another change really triggered her ire, "I don't like the way they are treating doctors these days. These young people don't respect them properly. When I trained, nurses gave total deference to doctors, giving up their seats at the desk and standing while awaiting their orders. All we ever said was 'Yes sir' or 'No sir.' We didn't question or make suggestions to them, ever."

Diagnosis and Hallelujahs

She remained upset throughout her training that doctors were no longer treated like royalty. Nurse Dixie made sure she always stood, awaiting orders, when one came to her station.

Back home after completing her training, her refrain changed to, "Now, what can I do? I can't work in one of the doctor's offices or be a floor nurse at Dad's hospital. It wouldn't be right. And what would people say if I went to work for any other medical center?"

Financially secure, Mom didn't need, nor want to work nine-to-five, fifty weeks of the year, but she needed to feel useful. Finally she figured it out.

"Oh Diane, exciting news. I've applied to be a camp nurse at Glorietta, that huge Baptist retreat in those gorgeous mountains in New Mexico. They have three on staff. I've been praying and this is what I think God wants me to do. I can't wait to hear from them."

We all waited to hear if Mom was going to camp.

"I'm hired. They want me." Only Dixie would consider taking on such a task at her age. She, who still napped every afternoon and hadn't worked in forty years, was going to be on shift rotation.

Upbeat and excited, off she went. Days went by and we didn't hear from her. A week later, while ironing, glancing up occasionally to watch a luxury cruise ship or freighter moving up Vancouver harbor, I heard the phone ring. Setting the iron down, I tossed Rex's damp shirt back in the plastic bag so it wouldn't dry out and hustled to the kitchen phone.

"Diane. It's your mother."

"Mom, how are you? What are you doing? How is camp?" I asked, alarmed at the weary tone of her voice.

"They tell me this is the roughest week, and I certainly hope so."

"Why? What's happened?"

"We have over 2,000 teenagers here—and they are all on skateboards. All I do all day long is patch up awful raw scrapes on elbows and knees and legs and sometimes heads where they have wiped out on these steep mountain roads. Otherwise, I love it. Of course my dorm room is too small. Really cramped. And the dorm is so noisy I have trouble sleeping and I don't have a private phone. But the people are really friendly."

With a voice becoming more and more animated, she added, "And I love the mountains, the pine trees, I even need a sweater at night. It's so much cooler than Texas. And I got my first paycheck. It wasn't very much. I took a few of the staffers out to dinner in Santa Fe last night and that wiped it all out."

Hmmmm. I hoped this rapid talk didn't indicate a manic episode. I had read that changes in schedules, especially sleep patterns, could trigger one. Should I ask her if she's still taking her lithium? If she lapses and starts having an episode, should I call the administration? And tell them what? I kept mum, but that didn't stop me from wondering about what would happen if she did stop those pills.

Whether it was a mild mania or Mom's zest for life, she soon became a popular person on campus. What amazed her the most was that her status was based on herself, not that she was Dr. Dweller's wife.

Welcome to the seventies, Mom.

Nurse Dixie went to camp for three summers. Each gave her unique memories she shared with us, like the time she was taken up to a campground on a mountainside in the middle of the night to help a camper who was having seizures. As she bent over him, his body went rigid, his feet kicked out, knocking Mom down. Over she went in a backward somersault, tumbling down the hillside several times, finally coming to a stop, fortunately, unhurt.

Gracie and I both went to see her when she returned home that third summer. After greeting us Mom said, "Come on girls, help me shell these peas." She led the way out to the backyard and we all settled down in lawn chairs, a gentle breeze making it pleasant in the late afternoon shade. She passed out newspapers and divided up the black-eyed pea pods among us. We started shelling. The peas made plopping sounds as they tumbled out of the shells onto the newspapers.

"You'll never guess what happened to me on the way back from Glorietta," Mom announced. With animated gestures and a vivacious voice, she embarked on her tale.

"I was driving out of the mountains and into the foothills, heading back home when I came over a hilltop and saw two police cruisers. They were blocking the highway. Their red lights were flashing. I almost couldn't stop without hitting them. I think they call it 'burning rubber.' The tire stench was awful." Mom fanned her nose with her hand, a pea pod in its grip.

Diagnosis and Hallelujahs

153

"A New Mexico trooper came running toward me with his hand on his gun." Mom glanced from Gracie to me, her eyes shining, obviously delighted to see our big-eyed responses. "At least it was still in his holster."

Shocked silent, my thoughts were racing faster than Mom's. She's off her lithium. How are we going to get her back on it? I glanced at Gracie. A knowing look passed between us.

Mom continued, "When I rolled down my window he looked surprised."

I bet he did. An older woman instead of some fugitive.

I asked him, "What's going on?"

She paused, lips in a pout. "He yelled at me. "This roadblock is for you! Do you have any idea how fast you've been going? A patrolman tried to catch you from behind and had to give up. He radioed ahead for us to try to stop you."

"How fast were you going Mom?" Gracie asked.

"I'm not telling," Mom replied with a lift of her chin.

"Did you get a ticket?"

"I sure did."

"How much was the ticket?"

"I'm not telling that either."

And she never did, no matter how many times we teasingly asked her over the years.

The questions I itched to ask, but didn't were: Did you decide to go off of lithium, or just run out? If you ran out of your prescription why didn't you get the Glorietta doctor to write one? What else did you do after you stopped your pills?

We never found out what else she did at Glorietta that summer, but the fact that she wasn't asked back the next summer gave us a clue that she probably went into a full blown manic episode that got the attention of the administration. The most important question now was: How can we get her to start taking lithium again?

Feeling timid, but desperate, I called Dr. Fisher and tattled on Mom, again. I don't know what magic he used to get her to start lithium again, but "hallelujahs" echoed through our house once more. Back on that little pill, Mom's rocket-speed behavior slowed down to normal—for a while.

15

Compliance Challenges

THE YEARS AFTER DAD'S DEATH brought changes to all our lives, especially Mom's. Both of my parents had loved traveling to exotic foreign places and Mom continued to travel abroad on group tours. She also played some bridge, but her daily activities often included helping others. An extrovert who enjoyed meeting new people, Mom became the Newcomers' Welcome Lady for her church. Other activities included visiting shut-ins every week plus helping with bereaved families.

While Mom adjusted to single life, Rex, the children and I were making major adjustments too. In 1977 we moved to Pennsylvania where Rex became a professor at a large university. I started job hunting only to discover the school districts were cutting back on the frills: art, music, and drama; thus, with my son heading to college that year and my older daughter in two years, I could not get an art teaching job. Maybe Dad was right: I should have majored in English or history.

As Rex had finished his advanced degrees only four years earlier, we faced a serious cash flow crisis. My best bet at making money fast turned out to be a real estate license. I took a crash course, read how-to books, passed my test, staked out my territory and started making cold calls door-to-door. Within a week I had my first listing and, surprising myself, managed to make enough money over the next two years to help send both kids to the universities of their choice.

Although successful as a real estate agent, I longed to do something that related to my art interest. Once more Gracie helped me. This time by arriving for a visit wearing a dark red dress.

"Hey, Gracie, over here," I called out as I spied her. "Wow, you look great in that red dress. I've never seen you wear anything red because of your

Compliance Challenges 155

auburn hair. How did you decide to buy it?"

"It's on my color chart."

"Your what?"

Gracie reached in her handbag and extracted a card holder full of a rainbow of colors, including the deep red brick color she was wearing. "I had a private consultation with a color consultant. These are the colors she tested on me that look good."

Fascinating. Looking at her in that red dress, I was sold. Thus as the fledgling personal image consulting industry started, I jumped on it, delighted to start a business where I could use my art training.

I made the mistake of telling Mom on the phone that I would be going to California to train as a color consultant. Her instant response, "Diane, that is the stupidest idea you've had yet. What makes you think anybody will ever pay you a dime to tell them what colors to wear?"

There was one constant I could still count on over the years—lithium or not—Mom's negative opinion about everything I did.

I went to training without her blessing.

Within a year, clients were waiting months to secure an appointment. And yes, they did pay me.

MOM CAME FOR A VISIT the next summer. Observing her interactions with Rex amused me. They had developed a wary relationship with Mom tiptoeing around topics that might tempt Rex to challenge her. It seemed ironic that Rex had no hesitations in dealing with Dixie, nor did I have any problem standing up to Rex's irascible father. But it appeared that coping mechanisms established in our childhoods followed both of us into adulthood, making it hard for each of us to alter deep-rooted reactions to our own parent. Rex did have a heated showdown with his dad years before I got up the courage to have my long-planned confrontation with Mom.

ONE FROSTY MORNING SEVERAL MONTHS after Mom's visit, I hurried out onto the wide porch of our three-story Victorian home and gathered several letters from our pedestal mail box. I shivered in the brisk wind that carried an acrid hint of the steel mills along the river. Hustling back inside, I sifted through the stack of mail and paused when I felt a thicker than usual letter from Mom.

Oh no. Not again. Please, not again.

Back in the kitchen I poured a second cup of coffee, headed into the sunroom and plopped down in my wicker rocking chair. Looking out at the bleak, leafless trees, I took several small sips of tongue-tingling hot coffee, trying to warm up and enjoy some tranquility before ripping open Mom's blue envelope.

My heart sank as two newspaper clippings fluttered to the hardwood floor. I stared in dismay at her first page. Each line of her handwriting, part cursive, part printing, slanted up the page toward the corner, its trajectory looking as if it were going to soar off the paper. As her scrawl continued, each line of script became smaller and smaller. Scribbled extra notes decorated the left and right margins. The three pages were filled with comments as jumbled as a child's toy box: Tues bridge. Jean forgot messed up everybody. Awful about Bob and Jenny. No explanation as to what was so awful. I didn't want to read the clear message between each of the lines. Mom had stopped her pills. Again.

Fortunately I knew who to call. "Dr. Fisher, have you seen my mother lately?"

"No, she keeps cancelling her appointments."

"Please contact her. She's evidently quit taking her lithium again."

About every eighteen months, Mom, feeling normal for a few months, declared she was cured and didn't need to take her medication anymore. She knew lithium needed to be taken daily, over time, to stabilize her mood swings. She knew, she knew, that every time she stopped it she had another manic episode. Yet off she went. Why? Why? WHY?

Needing to understand her maddening behavior better, I went to the nearby university medical school library. Perusing the latest research articles, I discovered Mom wasn't the only one shunning this wonder-working pill. An Australian study of bipolar patients who were followed for a year reported that over half were partially or totally non-compliant. And intermittent use of lithium increased the risk of episodes.

The more I read about the tragic lives, loves, jobs, families and financial security destroyed by this crazy chemical chaos called manic-depression or bipolar disorder, the more I realized how fortunate we were.

Mom's bipolar version, while totally irritating and frustrating, turned out not to be as aberrant as many others. She didn't buy five coffee pots or order six cute little golf carts like some people have done during their manic episodes.

Compliance Challenges 157

I read that not all bipolar patients exhibit the same symptoms, making bipolar disorder difficult to diagnose. And I learned Mom's superior attitude, called grandiosity, indicated she considered herself very important and she expected others to recognize her as such. It was her racing thoughts, fueled by sleeping only three or four hours each night during an episode, that drove her frantic actions. Unfortunately the brakes that usually curtailed unacceptable social actions also appeared to fail.

One article described a trait called "irritable mania," a variation that reveals itself with quick temper flashes, an impossibility to please and aggressive criticism of others. I reread that accurate description of Mom. Quick temper. Impossible to please. Aggressive criticism.

I could have written that description. I had lived it.

My self-esteem would have preferred the five coffee pots.

I felt cheated. Cheated out of a normal mother. All because of an erratic chemical in her brain I had a mother compelled to be irritable, impossible to please and who would continue to aggressively criticize me. Was there to be no end to this behavior?

Lithium did calm Mom's behavior. Within a few weeks of starting her pills her wild driving, spending sprees and incessant chattering disappeared, but not the constant criticisms. I wondered as I sat there—which of her traits were caused by her illness and which were caused by her basic personality? How intertwined were they?

My heart filled with sadness. Since those scary days of childhood, I had harbored the hope that one day Mom would show me some sign of affection—hug me, or tell me that she loved me. Did her chemical imbalance mean this would never happen? If we could get her to stay on lithium would she stop criticizing me? Would she ever become more loving?

I slid back in the wooden library chair and stared across the room, pondering these questions. If she stayed on her pills long enough, maybe, maybe, I mused, she would become more affectionate.

Dream on Diane.

I turned back to the journals and books scattered on the long table in front of me. While Mom's behavior disrupted our lives, it didn't come close to what some families experience. The most important aspect of Mom's version of manic-depression turned out to be her lack of depression.

Each time she declared, "I'm well," and stopped her pills, she blasted off into mania. The lifelong game she played between the two emotional goal posts resulted in a score of Manic Episodes, about 50, to only 1 for Depressive Episodes.

Aside from that one deep depression, we were spared the heartache of depressive cycles and suicide scares. It must be horrendous to fear that a family member may kill himself. Or to try to stop them from a life on illegal drugs or having sex with anyone, anyplace. Or spending the family resources into bankruptcy. My heart ached for these other families.

I tried to be thankful, but I couldn't totally pull that off. Every time Dr. Fisher convinced Mom to restart her lithium pills, the metronome started ticking, ticking. It would be just a matter of time until she stopped. Again.

As I HEADED BACK HOME, my tummy announced with a growl that it was way past lunchtime. I stopped in at a popular deli and treated myself to a Philly Cheesesteak sandwich with caramelized onions, sautéed green peppers and melted provolone cheese. Carrying my tray, I found an empty table next to the window. I munched, sipped coffee, people-watched and tapped my foot to the background music. A lively polka evoked a long-ago image of Mom laughing and dancing a polka on the top of Lookout Mountain. It brought a grin to my face. Manic Mom did know how to have a good time.

While we all have our own unique dance moves, as a manic episode progressed Mom danced to many different tempos. As it began, she would move in a peppy polka-like pace—having a wonderful time, happy, laughing, hyper-focused and productive. As her thoughts accelerated, it was more like trying to keep up with "Dueling Banjos," as first one idea and then another propelled her hectic actions. Her inner rhythm buzzed even into the midnight hours when she would bang the iron onto the board with a ferocity that reverberated through the house. The peak of an episode exploded like the fireworks of Tchaikovsky's "1812 Overture," with bursts of clashing cymbals, firing cannons and tirades of negative comments. Her melt-down tempo was symbolic of a Bartok composition, with broken, silent pauses and sometimes dissonant chords as she ignored the impact of her actions and words and returned to her version of normal behavior.

She never, ever, it appeared, heard a lullaby.

Compliance Challenges

At the end of each manic episode Mom acted like nothing unusual had transpired during the previous weeks. I wondered if memories of her behavior disappeared like rocks thrown into a pond, after creating the ripples that tossed her—and our—lives around.

Neither Gracie nor I ever talked to Mom about anything weird she did during an episode. Breathing a sigh of relief that another spell had ended became our way of coping and avoiding more unpleasantness by confronting her. We acted like that spell never happened.

We had herds of elephants in our living rooms.

A FEW WEEKS LATER, BROWSING in a bookstore, I came across a book titled *An Unquiet Mind, A Memoir of Moods and Madness* by Dr. Kay Redfield Jamison. A professor of psychiatry at The Johns Hopkins School of Medicine, Jamison is an internationally recognized medical expert on bipolar disorder. She also knows what manic-depression is like from the inside-out, as she suffers from it herself.

Jamison described herself at a faculty garden party as "irresistibly charming" and "captivating." The faculty member, who later became her psychiatrist, recalled her looking "wild-eyed, frenzied, far too talkative and manic."

Like Jamison, Mom, also appeared to think she was the life of the party and her ideas and actions were terrific during her manic episodes.

Jamison's statement that "mania has at least some grace in partially obliterating memories" confirmed my suspicions that if we ever did confront Mom about her behavior during a manic episode, her recall would probably be different from ours—and from reality.

RECEIVING INCOMPREHENSIBLE LETTERS FROM MOM wasn't the only clue she was experiencing another bout of mania. An excited phone call from her rang even louder alarm bells. By the time she called, she would be soaring and aggravating everyone from the preacher to her hairdresser. Something dramatic always occurred—like canceling health insurance, firing yard help, crunching another fender, moving again or buying another car.

We were fortunate to feel free to call Dr. Fisher when we needed his help. Mom's respect for doctors helped him get her back on track time and again. Until she again declared, "I'm well."

To me, one of the mysteries about bipolar disorders is the months of normal behavior between either manic or depressive episodes that occur for most patients. Why, and how, does that happen? It was often during those normal days that Mom declared herself cured and stopped that magic little pill—again.

Gracie and I did not understand why she kept doing this. Didn't she want to stay normal? Jamison's revelations helped us again:

> "Once I felt well again I had neither the desire nor incentive to continue with medicine ... I missed my highs; and once I felt normal again, it was very easy for me to deny that I had an illness that would come back. Somehow I was convinced that I was an exception to the extensive research literature, which clearly showed not only that manic-depressive illness comes back, but that it often comes back in a more severe and frequent form."

EACH TIME MOM STOPPED HER pills her mania came roaring back, usually in about a month.

One research paper reported this was to be expected. Lithium would not cure her chemical imbalance, just stabilize it. The fact that this medication reduced Mom's manic spells confirmed she was bipolar and that she needed to take it. Like the tiny puffs of air used to stabilize the yaw of a huge space craft speeding through the heavens, that tiny lithium pill stabilized Mom's speeding thoughts and actions. Smart enough to understand this, Mom was too stubborn or too selfish—missing her highs—to keep taking that magic potion.

Each time she provoked another manic episode, I felt relief that I now lived so far away. At least at a distance I didn't have to see how people were reacting to her behind her back.

Each time I wondered, what is my responsibility to this woman, this mother who gave me life? I felt hopeless exasperation. It was bad enough before we knew what caused her spells. Now that we knew lithium stabilized her brain chemistry, her choice to stop her prescription became totally unacceptable.

When other bipolar patients repeatedly stop their medications, I suspect their families, like ours, become disgusted and angry that their relative is

Compliance Challenges

161

not complying. Stopping this vital medication affects everyone in contact with the erring patient—family, friends, co-workers and even strangers.

Gracie and I conferred, trying to come up with ideas on how to stop this repeated cycle. They were short conversations. Nothing seemed to work. Chiding her didn't. Nor begging. The anticipation of what she might do during her next manic episode kept us on tenterhooks.

Mom kept playing pill-roulette. She never appeared to consider the impact of her behavior on Gracie or me. Each time she instigated another manic episode I didn't just feel disgusted, I wanted OUT. I wanted to divorce her, to be rid of her and her problem, but I knew I couldn't leave Gracie to deal with her alone. Nevertheless, frustrated by this recurring scenario, we both wanted to know how to cancel our reserved seats on Dixie's next space odyssey.

BESIDES NONSENSICAL LETTERS OR FRANTIC phone calls, another solid clue that Mom was on-or-off her lithium showed up in her gifts. Before lithium, no one could be more generous with money when she was manic, nor parsimonious when not. My older daughter Andrea seemed to always catch a penny-pinching period for her birthday.

On Andrea's tenth birthday, Mom's gift arrived in a beautiful store-wrapped box with shiny paper and pink bow. Andrea eagerly tore into the package. As she lifted off the top of the white box and pulled back the tissue paper, her face registered confusion. Inside was a multicolored square neck scarf like an old lady would wear—not anything a ten-year-old would like, want or ever consider wearing.

Several years later, teenaged Andrea looked even less excited when she slowly opened her Grandmother's gift to reveal several too-big blouses— Mom's old blouses, still reeking of White Shoulders perfume. What could Mom have been thinking? This gift should have been sent to a charity, not to a granddaughter on her birthday. And why did she think her grandsons would want a kettle to boil water? Our family started making a game of guessing what weird item would be in her gift boxes: dried or plastic flowers, fruit cake, glass shelving or figurines from her travels.

I didn't comment to Mom about how disappointing her bizarre gifts were. She always had a reason or excuse for her weird actions, like, "Of course the boys need to know how to boil water."

As the grandchildren matured, fortunately Mom started giving birthday and Christmas checks instead of strange items. One year we were flabbergasted to open her gift cards and discover checks for $10,000 each.

Guess who was manic.

The next Christmas my niece said it all when she looked at her $100 check and asked, "Aren't there some zeros missing?"

Recipients of Mom's parsimony that never wavered, manic times or not, were the unfortunate waiters who were lucky to get even a two dollar tip for excellent service on a very expensive meal. One of us always stayed behind at the table to rectify her adamant refusal to tip better.

Prior to her diagnosis, Mom's episodes occurred randomly, lasting for weeks each time. While some patients have seasonal episodes, I never observed a systematic timing of hers. Trauma, like the death of her baby and later her husband, threw her into manic mode. Now the episodes were only triggered when she stopped her pills.

Being manic enticed Mom, promising fun and excitement. Being normal must have seemed like a depression compared to her exuberant feelings during mania. And who would choose dull, boring normal when all you have to do to soar into your own exciting orbit is stop taking a pill.

Like most families of people who are bipolar, we lived with a constant undercurrent of uneasiness, always wondering how long it would be until that proverbial other shoe dropped. Then the next one . . . and the next.

16

Sad Anger:
Confrontation # 3

C LEANING UP THE BREAKFAST DISHES early one morning I heard the phone ring. Alarm bells started ringing in my head. Who else would be calling before seven in the morning? What has she done now?

I reached around the sunroom doorway, grabbed the receiver off the wall phone and said, "Hello Mom."

"Oh Diane, I'm having the best time and I sold our house last night."

"Sold the house?" Needing to sit down all of a sudden, I sank down on the step to the sunroom before asking, "When did you decide to sell it?"

"Four days ago," she continued in an excited voice, "and I had a date. With Ted Hightower. I had a dinner party and asked him to be my date and he accepted. We went to the Steak House and joined three more couples I invited. And oh, he liked my blonde hair. You know they say blondes have more fun and I think they do. I'm having so much fun I even bought a full-length mink coat. It's gorgeous, dark brown and so soft. I love it. Don't want to take it off."

"Let me get this straight," I said in a weak voice, "this week, you sold the house you and dad built, that you've lived in for thirty years? You called Ted for a date, arranged a dinner party, bleached your hair blonde and bought a mink coat?"

She laughed with glee and added, "And I forgot to tell you about the coffee. Loads of fun. Had sixteen friends over Tuesday morning."

My thoughts whirled. She had sold our home. I had no idea she ever planned to sell our family home.

"Where do you plan to live?" I asked.

"I don't know. I'll find something later after I get back from Austin."

"Why are you going to Austin?"

"Jean belongs to the Federated Women's Club and I'm going with her to their state convention."

"But you don't even belong to a Federated Women's club."

GOOD GRIEF. WHAT WOULD SHE do next? I had no clue until that phone call that Mom had stopped her lithium. It had been almost two years since she had last stopped her medication and gone into a manic episode. Obviously she had done it again—big time, this time.

After I hung up the phone, I sat there a long time looking out at my garden. As the sun rose I watched the sunbeams shining between the branches of our huge maple trees slowly move across the bay window. Even this tranquil scene couldn't unsnarl the knots in my stomach, the helplessness in my heart.

Did Mom ever want to be normal? Evidently not. Once again she challenged fate and once again Gracie and I would have to try and get her back on that pill and undo any financial damage. She would have to repair her own social life.

I felt exhausted, tired of trying to deal time and again with the most obstinate woman God ever created, tired of living under the threat of her doing things in a manic whirl, like selling her house and buying mink coats.

Why don't I look her in the eye and tell her, "Go ahead, stop your lithium, speed-drive, have wrecks, kill someone, alienate your friends, spend yourself into poverty." Why? Because she wouldn't hear it, heed it or change. I wish now I had kept records and data each time she stopped her medication, including how soon her next manic episode started, how long it lasted. Confronting her during a normal period with the data of the strange decisions she made during it, her expenditures, her speeding tickets and bizarre behavior might have kept her on lithium—or at least on it for longer periods. Maybe.

I called Gracie with the house news.

"She sold the house?" Her shocked tone resonated through the phone. After I related the list of Mom's frantic activities, I heard only silence. Then sighing, she asked, "What else can we do to convince her that she has to stay on lithium? Pleading hasn't worked. Or anger. Or prayers. Nothing has."

How fortunate we knew Dr. Fisher. What would Gracie and I have done without him?

Sad Anger: Confrontation # 3

I called him and said. "I suspect Dixie has cancelled her appointments lately."

"Yes, the last two."

"Would you please contact her? Her behavior is off the charts." I explained what she had been up to in the past six days, ending with, "Don't be surprised when a blonde walks in wearing a mink coat. It will be Dixie."

The next month I joined Gracie in helping Mom move. By that time, back on lithium, she had settled down—somewhat—and become a brunette again.

It was fascinating to see what Mom had given away, sold and kept by the time I got there. Vintage items to be moved included outdated thirty-year-old Compton Encyclopedias and her oversized phonograph player. Gracie stared at it, hands on her hips, but then with a grin started looking through the large records. Selecting several, she put on a stack of 78s and we started packing towels and linens to Lena Horn belting out *Stormy Weather*.

Gone were many things Gracie and I wanted, like the movies of us as babies and toddlers.

"But," Mom exclaimed shaking her head, "they don't make projectors for that size reels anymore and I didn't know you could get them transferred to other film,"

Gracie said, "I wish you had asked before you threw them away. I do hope you kept all those wonderful sympathy cards and letters from patients who wrote to tell us how wonderful Dad was."

"Oh I threw all those away right after the funeral."

I CONTINUED TO LIMIT MY trips to North Creek. Mom occasionally visited us; other years we met in Dallas at Gracie's home, or at Granny's farm.

On my last visit to the farm, Granny proudly walked me through her old house, pointing out specific items some of her descendants wanted to inherit—her oak sideboard with the mirror, her butter churn, an antique trunk.

I hesitated, then recalling the doll quilts Mom had thrown away when we were children, I asked, "A quilt. Granny, would you please put my name on a quilt you made."

Visiting Granny's as an adult helped me comprehend how challenging it must have been during Mom's childhood before they had modern conveniences like running water. Her childhood, laced with hard physical labor and embarrassment over her low economic status probably became the basis for her fear of what people would say. It may have contributed to her demands that we always do things so properly—and her frustrations when we didn't.

Seeing each other at Granny's or Gracie's didn't satisfy Mom. She wanted me to come home. Of course, to me, the word "home" meant the house she sold. Visiting her in a different apartment each visit wasn't the same. And who wants to go see someone who constantly criticizes you anyway?

"Can't you come home?" Mom wrote and asked for the umpteenth time.

I called her. "Mom, it costs as much to travel from Pennsylvania to North Creek as it would cost to go to Paris, France. Why don't we meet there?" I hoped this idea would strike her love-to-travel chord and a different environment might keep me from feeling trapped in our past relationship. Nothing doing. She insisted I come home to her latest apartment.

Feeling guilty, at last I relented. Shannon, now ten, and I headed to hot Texas.

"Good grief," I exclaimed as I stepped out of the plane onto the tarmac and felt the wind whipping my hair into my face at such a furious pace that it stung. No wonder Texas women were still wearing super-sprayed, back-combed, bee-hive hair styles in 1982. I reached up to hold my flying locks in place, very thankful that the wind didn't have any sand in it.

"Hey Diane, Shannon. Over here," Mom waved, then frowned as she looked up and down at what I wore. I had on a raw silk dress that showed my figure to an advantage and matched my now auburn highlights that disguised those relentless strands of gray that started showing up in my twenties. While I had received more than one unsolicited compliment when wearing this outfit, Mom didn't have to say anything to communicate that she didn't like it. It wasn't an intensely bright color like the bright yellow polyester slacks she had on nor her exploding multicolored flowered top.

The drive from the airport to North Creek revealed a dry spell with puny cotton plants, stunted and wilting in the hot sun. It looked as desolate as I remembered. Not at all like Paris.

Mom chatted while I drove. "I've planned a coffee tomorrow morning for all your friends in the area." That surprised me. Very thoughtful. Looking

Sad Anger: Confrontation # 3

forward to visiting with my girlfriends, I reconsidered that maybe this trip would be different. But as that day progressed, so did Mom's critiques of me. Irritated, I bit back retorts, trying to shrug them off. Then I got mad at myself for allowing her to do this to me once more.

Why do I still react to her criticisms? I know to expect them. Why am I still reacting like a child? Grow up Diane. You don't have to put up with her criticisms anymore. Tell her to stop. Tell her off.

I sat there silently making excuses, the same old excuses to myself: It won't do any good to try and stop her. She will never stop mothering, criticizing or correcting me.

Mom's latest apartment turned out to be larger than her last one. The two story interior was drowning in beige from top to bottom: beige walls, beige carpet, beige appliances, beige bathrooms. The only touches of home to me were her ever-present favorite turquoise sofa plus a jungle that now consisted of plastic, artificial houseplants.

BLURP. BLURP-BLURP. SOUNDS FROM THE percolator emanated from the kitchen as the time of the morning party approached; the smell of freshly brewed coffee soon filled the air.

While dusting the coffee table and beige lamps as Mom directed, I heard Shannon in the kitchen ask if she could cut the lemon pound cake Mom had baked in her Bundt cake pan.

"Okay," I heard Mom reply.

Several minutes of silence followed, then a horrified, shrill scream, "NO, NO, NO. YOU'VE RUINED THE CAKE. OH MY LANDS. DON'T YOU KNOW HOW TO SLICE A CAKE? IT'S RUINED. RUINED. YOU'RE SUPPOSED TO CUT IT IN THE VALLEYS. OH DEAR, IT'S RUINED. ALL THAT WORK."

I hurried into the kitchen. My heart fell when I saw Shannon's face, her bottom lip trembling. Immediately I became a child again, feeling the terror of Mom's instant screaming tirades. Rage consumed me as memories of Scary Mom flashed through my mind. I hugged Shannon, struggling to contain my anger in front of her. What I really wanted to do was scream at Mom.

Instead, I took a deep breath and struggled to say calmly, "It isn't ruined Shannon, and Grandmother should have shown you how she wanted it cut. I'll fix it."

"No, I'll do it," Mom barked, grabbing the knife off the counter. She fumed, "All that work, ruined, ruined. I could cry." Just as we turned to leave her in the kitchen, the doorbell rang. The guests had arrived.

The entire rest of the day, my thoughts tumbled, my anger grew.

That night, before crawling into the guestroom bed, I called Rex, seething about the cake incident. "Mom is treating Shannon like she treated me. I'm beyond furious. I don't see how I am going to stay here another five days without exploding."

While I couldn't find the backbone to stand up to Mother's constant criticism of me all these years, my instinct to protect my child after her grandmother's tirade consumed me. Enough. I seethed, tossing and turning for hours, mad, not only at Mom but at myself for not confronting her. I swore to myself—she's never going to scream at Shannon like that again.

I thought I had purged my ire toward Mom years ago with all that flushing, burning and stamping on my bad memories. Rather than totally eliminating those negative feelings, it appeared I had pushed them down into the core of a dormant volcano where they had been smoldering all these years. Those embers now burst into flames, shooting flares of painful memories back into my consciousness—whippings, criticisms, her reaction to my divorce, that damn letter, her constant put-downs about my appearance, my career . . .

As usual, my lifelong litany of confrontations with Mom happened only in my mind. I started imagining the showdown we would have the next day. I would tear into her, lambasting her with scathing words, cutting words, ugly words, hurtful words—words that told her what an awful mother she had been. I imagined saying:

Do you think buying me clothes and taking me to plays as a child wiped out the horrible whippings, or made up for not hugging me? Never giving me one compliment, or one thank you for a job well done, or even one word of encouragement?

Do you think anything can ever erase all the times you've criticized me . . . never enough A's on a report card . . . my hair always looks awful. . .everything I do fails to meet your impossible expectations. I'm sorry I have thin hair, that I'm not pretty. That I shamed you when I got a divorce. That I'm not perfect. But aren't mothers supposed to love their children despite their bad hair, their failed marriage or the shape of their finger nails?

Sad Anger: Confrontation # 3

I can't stand to be around you another day. Nor do I want Shannon to hear you constantly criticizing me either. We're leaving.

With that thought, I got out of the bed and started throwing my clothes back into the suitcase. That didn't take long. Who cared if they got wrinkled? Not me.

Sitting back down on the bed, I grabbed the pillow, beat it into shape, threw it back on the bed and flopped down, staring at the ceiling. Teeth clamped. Looking up, I noticed daylight starting to show around the edges of the beige draperies.

Sleep still elusive, I lay there vowing not to let another day of my life go by without standing up to her.

That morning started like others—Mom still critical, me still silently taking it. Not wanting to have a showdown in front of Shannon, I kept biding my time, still not sure how or when I would unload forty-plus years of pent-up anger at Mom. All morning I felt my stomach churning. Bile, tasting of bacon, irritated my throat.

Late morning, the three of us went upstairs to our respective bedrooms to change clothes before meeting some of Mom's friends for lunch. As I finished trying to fluff my hair up more I heard Shannon going down the stairs and the television come on.

Mom and I came out of our bedrooms onto the upstairs landing at the same time. She looked me up and down, then stated in a derogatory tone, "You aren't wearing that, are you?"

I stared at her for a long moment, rage instantly bubbling. Caustic retorts jumped into my mind. I opened my mouth to let them out. But something deep inside of me snapped my mouth shut.

Instead of erupting in anger, spewing forth all those well-rehearsed barbs, I felt a calmness invade my head, quelling my rage, traveling down my entire body, similar to that cold rage I felt the time I confronted my ex-husband. Only this time it wasn't cold rage, but an overwhelming sadness.

No anger exploded. Instead, looking Mom in the eye, I announced in a very quiet, very firm tone, "That's it. No more. That is the last criticism you're allowed this trip."

"What do you mean?" she retorted.

"Since we woke up this morning you have criticized me four times."

"I have not."

I recalled each one, "You think my hair style is tacky, my career is frivolous, you don't approve of my letting Andrea go to college in Austin and now you don't like my outfit."

She could not deny she said each of those things.

Still amazing myself with my own calm, it seemed I almost stood outside of my body. I saw my arms reach out and gently surround her as I softly continued, "I came here hoping to have a good time with you, to go home with some good memories of our visit, but I can't do that when you constantly criticize me—or when you scream at Shannon. If you continue to criticize me or raise your voice at her again, we will leave."

Tightening my arms, I gave her now rigid body a soft hug, then turned and walked down the stairs. I got almost to the landing before my knees buckled. I held onto the banister the rest of the way down. Then my chin started to quiver. I sank down on the turquoise sofa, sucking in deep breaths. Where had that calmness come from? Those conciliatory words? And my reaching out to hug her? Our last hug had occurred when Dad died over nine years ago.

Taking another shaky breath, I realized I had finally done what I had wanted to do for over forty years. I looked Mom in the eye and told her to stop criticizing me. Demanded that she stop. Gave her a consequence if she didn't.

How sad that it took another crisis with one of my children for me to find the courage to do what I should have done years ago. My quivering lips began to turn up in a grin. A surge of glee washed over me. I did it. I finally challenged my challenging mom.

Some time elapsed before Mom came downstairs. We left for lunch with an awkwardness between us, without referring to the confrontation. For the next five days I saw her open her mouth, time and again, and start to say something, only to close it. She remained unusually quiet. I think, until then, she had no idea how often she criticized me.

What would have happened to our relationship if I had erupted in anger? Spewed all those pent-up ugly comments? Would an irreparable split have occurred? Thank heavens those surprising words of reconciliation came out of my mouth instead. That calm confrontation became a turning point

Sad Anger: Confrontation # 3

in our relationship. At forty-three I finally grew up and stopped enabling Mom to continue her verbal abuse.

Did Mom criticize me in the future? Of course. She never learned to stop mothering. But when her comments started getting to me, all I had to do was look her in the eye, smile and say, "Enough criticisms, Mom." She got my message each time.

Now the main obstacle to a tranquil life with Dixie consisted of trying to figure out how to keep her on that pill.

17

Doing Something Right

LATE ONE AFTERNOON WHILE TIDYING up my office, the phone starting ringing. I answered with my business greeting, followed by, "How may I help you?"

"Hi. It's your mother and I have some good news. Are you sitting down?"

I blew out a huff of air and with a sinking feeling plopped down in my office chair, not eager to hear what calamity her good news might be.

"I'm sitting. What's up?"

"I'm taking all of the family on a Caribbean cruise for a week." I blinked. That was good news, even if it meant she might be flying high while we were cruising.

Gracie's family of five joined our five and Mom in Miami during the summer school break for our holiday aboard a floating hotel with its multiple activities. Cha-cha music had all of us swaying to the beat as we walked up the gangplank—the five grandchildren ranging in age from eighteen to twenty-two, ten-year-old Shannon, and Mom who would turn seventy-three that November.

That cruise as a family created a wonderful memory of Mom. We ate meals together, laughing and sharing what we had been doing; otherwise, we went our separate ways, participating in many different activities on and off the ship. Our extended family team even won the island sand sculpture contest with a large sea dragon bejeweled with seaweed. Dixie, in a joyous mood the whole trip, flirted with every available man, and for once, suspended criticism for almost the entire week.

I finally asked her, "May I assume since you haven't critiqued anything I'm wearing that I look okay?"

"Well, you could use more lipstick."

Doing Something Right 173

MOM'S GENEROSITY DIDN'T END WITH the cruise. She decided to help all her grandchildren through college with a monthly check. This was totally unexpected. We were floored, and thankful. It was more than welcome. Our onerous total of college costs for two children continued to create a challenge for us financially, especially on an associate professor's salary. Every dollar I made in those days went to pay for their educations.

Mom kept up her end of the offer, sending checks to the five grandchildren until they all graduated in the next few years. She even set up a college fund for Shannon in case anything happened to her before her last grandchild went to college.

Gracie expressed dismay that the amount for Shannon totaled considerably less than Mom had given her older grandchildren. Mom's rationale: "It's going to earn interest and by the time Shannon goes to college in eight years it will equal the amount." Gracie tried to get her to understand that college costs were escalating yearly and the amount would not begin to be equal. Once Mom's mind fixated on a decision, it became unchangeable. She remained one stubborn lady. I was thrilled that she contributed anything. As frustrated as I could be with her at times, she never ceased to amaze me.

LATE ONE EVENING, REX AND I were watching a favorite television program in the upstairs sitting room, the warmth of a fire making the room feel cozy and calm. Suddenly the jarring ring of the phone broke the mood.

"Rex, turn down the TV please," I asked as I reached for the phone on the table between our easy chairs.

I answered, wondering who would be calling at this time of night.

"Diane, I just got back from Granny's," Mom's weary voice announced. "Mother died and we buried her Thursday."

"WHAT? Granny died? When?" Rex's head jerked around. I stood up, trying to catch my breath, to comprehend what I had heard. Disbelief flooded my head, my heart. *Not my Granny.*

"Last Monday," Mom replied.

"Why didn't you call me?"

"I didn't want you to feel like you had to come to the funeral," Mom explained.

174   MOM, MANIA, AND ME

Stunned speechless, I felt betrayed. Bewildered. Angry. Furious. I croaked out, "That should have been my decision, not yours."

My beloved Granny, Mom's own mother died and she decided not to tell me. How do you have closure, say a final goodbye or mend your heartache when every time you think about your Granny the main emotion you feel is anger at your mother?

Once again Mom believed that her ideas, opinions and actions were right. She thought she knew what was best for everyone, especially me. Wrong. Painful. Heartbreaking wrong.

Mom did send me the quilt Granny had put my name on. It is queen sized with a huge Texas Star pattern in the middle surrounded by a vivid blue background. A true treasure.

THE DISTANCE FROM PENNSYLVANIA TO Texas limited our family visits to about one per year when we would make the long two-day drive across half of the United States. On one visit to Gracie's home in Dallas, we two were enjoying some sister time alone in her cozy office lined with overflowing bookcases. Sitting in the gold recliner that had once been Mom's, I relaxed until our conversation turned to her latest antics. With a serious tone Gracie said, "Mother has done something awful. I hope you won't get too upset."

My relaxed mood evaporated as Gracie disappeared in the direction of her utility room. What could she be getting? Not sure what to expect, I felt every part of my body tense up while waiting to hear about Mom's latest fiasco. Gracie came back holding a small picture frame close to her chest. "Now don't be too mad, but I can't believe she ruined your painting like this." She handed me the first oil painting I ever did. I took one look at it and burst out laughing.

All those years ago Mom had insisted that if she were going to pay for art lessons, my first painting had to include some roses and a poem she loved. The verse by Frank L. Stanton stated:

This world that we're a livin' in

Is mighty hard to beat

You get a thorn with every rose

But ain't the roses sweet!

I had dutifully painted it exactly as it read. Only now my amateurish roses and lettering had big black ink scratches through the word "ain't" with the

Doing Something Right 175

word "aren't" inked in below it on the oil painting.

It hangs in my studio today, and every time I look at it, I chuckle. It is just so Dixie-like. Even my oil painting failed to get past her need to correct me, the poem—and the poet.

THE YEAR SHANNON TURNED ELEVEN, our core family of three spent the summer exploring Scotland. We bunked in a student dorm at a university located among the hills and dales near the charming village of Stirling. Every morning we were awakened at five o'clock by the screeching and groaning of a bagpiper practicing Scotland's version of music while marching on the local golf course. Didn't that piper know that those bleats that sounded like donkeys braying could be heard for blocks?

While Rex worked at the University of Strathclyde, Shannon and I spent fun days exploring Stirling Castle and poking our noses into the quaint butchers, bakers and glass-makers shops. I signed my tall pre-teen daughter up for modeling classes plus kayak lessons in the frigid waters of a nearby lock. Shannon and her mates shared the waterfront with a graceful mother swan who marred her elegant image by making nasty hissing sounds at the kayakers as she led her line of six tiny cygnets to safety.

As the summer ended, we changed our travel plans. We took several days meandering our way to London, not thinking to inform the relatives back in the states. Upon arrival at our hotel, we had a cryptic message from my niece who was studying in London. "Call home. Grandmother has cancer."

Cancer? What kind of cancer? How bad? I didn't know where to reach my niece for the details. Because the time difference made it two o'clock in the morning in Texas, I waited four very long hours before trying to call Gracie. My emotions tumbled in all directions. Had the cancer spread? Was Mom terminally ill? Please not. I still had unfinished emotional issues I needed to resolve with her. I tried to reach Gracie again. Totally frustrated after multiple transatlantic calls didn't get an answer, I finally called the hospital in North Creek and asked for Mrs. Dweller's room. They rang. Mom answered.

"Mom, it's Diane. How are you? What has happened? What kind of cancer do you have? Where is it? How bad is it?

"I'm fine. I just had colon cancer." Bad news. It ran in the family.

"What cancer treatments are planned? Will you have chemo and radiation?"

"No, I had cancer. The surgery got it all. I don't have to have any more treatments. I'm going home today. I'm fine," she said. Her blithe responses struck me as weird. She reacted to my not having on lipstick or Shannon not cutting a Bundt shaped cake in the creases as a horrific calamity, but having cancer appeared to be just an inconvenience.

Once again my brain was baffled by the way her brain worked.

THAT SUMMER, ANDREA, NEEDING TO pick up some extra college credits, went to live with her grandmother and take the courses at the junior college I had attended. It didn't go smoothly.

"Mom," she exploded over the phone soon after her arrival, "Grandmother is driving me crazy. She criticizes everything I wear and she wants me to wear a GIRDLE. How did you and Gracie ever turn out normal?"

I'm not sure we did.

LATER, A LETTER FROM ANDREA revealed that a different perception of her fun Grandmother had begun to emerge.

> Grandmother is trying so hard to help that sometimes I wish she wouldn't. It's not so much that she wants to help that bothers me, it's that she does it without asking me. Whatever <u>she</u> feels is "best" for me she dives in . . .
>
> I say no thank you, no thank you, no thank you and she says yes, yes, yes!

During that summer Andrea sustained serious cuts on her upper arm in an auto accident that required an ambulance and stitches, plus major auto repairs. Her letter, written the week after the accident, reveals her account of her grandmother's manic mood swing.

> Grandmother and I had two very stormy arguments over her actions and reactions to all of this. Fri-Sun I didn't feel like even thinking about it and so she went berserk calling all over town about what to do and when she wasn't doing that she was complaining and <u>WORRYING</u> OUT LOUD to me 24 hrs. a day. It really upset me even more—having

Doing Something Right 177

to deal with Dixie on top of everything else just put the icing on the cake. I mean from the time she woke-up (<u>literally</u>) at breakfast she'd be looking over the phone book to find body-repair shops or salvage places until bed time and then she told me she had been waking up in the middle of the night Fri., Sat., Sun worrying over what to do.

"No matter what I say/do she thinks I'm incompetent and wants to ask someone else what <u>they</u> think or she tells me what I "<u>should</u>" do—it seems very unlike her to get this out-of-shape. I finally blew up at her one night and told her that (1) <u>I</u> was going to handle everything from here on out, (2) that <u>I</u> would do things when I want, the way I want to do them!

HURRAY FOR ANDREA. SHE STOOD up to Mom. Andrea was very capable of taking care of the entire situation, but unfortunately I knew that Mom would fret out loud endlessly before deciding what would be done, irrespective of Andrea's wishes. I knew Andrea's confrontation would not stop Mom, but at least standing up to her kept Andrea from being a wimp like me.

MY BUSINESS CONTINUED TO FLOURISH. My motivation to excel remained firmly tied to my driving desire to succeed in spite of, or because of, Mom's negative comments about my career choice. Mom didn't ask about my business, nor did I discuss it with her, having heard how stupid I was to become an image consultant.

The reasons one chooses a certain career path are not always clear, but Mom's hundreds of critical comments about my appearance finally paid off. During the years of living at home I had learned to scrutinize everything about my appearance every day, from hairstyle to shoes, not expecting a compliment, but in hopes of not being criticized. Her criticisms made me super-aware of the impact different combinations of clothes and accessories could make on my body. Even at age eleven, before my spinal surgery, I noticed certain garments made my body look more lopsided, while others appeared to conceal my curvature. These insights trained my eye to see the impact of the lines and shape of a garment on a female figure years before my art training taught me about form, balance and proportion.

I often heard from my clients, "What styles are best for me?" They often expressed negative feelings about their bodies: my hips, my bosom, my skinny legs, my tummy . . . They wanted advice about finding clothing that would enhance their bodies. Stumped about what to advise them, I began collecting information. The books stacked up in a corner of my office until, laid up with a health problem for several weeks, I started trying to figure out answers to their questions.

Once I became mobile, I headed to a nearby spa with my tape measure to try out my ideas on real women. I soon learned two things: I didn't like measuring women, and, they didn't like to be measured. At last, after days of trial and error, I came up with a unique way to evaluate a woman's body proportions without measurements. Using visual aids, a woman's body proportions could easily be observed without knowing how much she weighed or how many inches her hips actually were.

I created a few handouts with some guidelines and sketches for my clients. When some of my image colleagues saw them, I started hearing, "May I have a copy?" The word spread. Requests increased. A light bulb went off. Maybe I should put all this information in a chart and start charging for it.

Over the next year I sat at my drafting table and computer often, loving every minute of the challenging evolution of my ideas. After obtaining a hard-to-get business loan, my large chart, plus an instructor's manual for image consultants to use in classes, rolled off the presses. The consultant's feedback: "Everyone loves your system but we all dislike trying to fold up this large chart. Can you turn this into a smaller workbook?" After making the layout revisions, back to the printer I went. I also had to go back to the bank, this time borrowing enough money to market my workbook nationally.

During the next couple of years I gained a reputation as an entertaining national speaker with my demonstrations on volunteers from the audience. After speaking at the national convention for home economics teachers, I made the rounds of the book booths asking the representatives who they would recommend to publish an expanded version of my workbook. One exhibitor gave me the name of a personal contact at a major publisher. Back in my office, I sent off a copy of the workbook with a letter spelling out my goals and current success.

Several months later, actually having been so busy I had forgotten about

Doing Something Right

my letter, the phone in my home office rang.

I answered, "Diane Dweller's office. Diane speaking."

"Are you the author of a workbook about helping women select clothes?"

"Yes, I am. How may I help you?

She identified herself as an editor at the large publishing firm. "We have received a copy of your workbook and we are interested in your ideas for a consumer book. Do you have a minute?"

Did I ever. I bolted upright, sitting tall, all senses zinging. The lively discussion occurring over the next hour concluded with an arrangement for us to meet in two weeks at their headquarters in New York City. I hung up the phone and sat there a full minute. Did what just happened, really happen? As the reality hit me I jumped out of my chair and into the air letting loose a loud "WHOOPIE."

I called everyone who cared, especially Rex, who had encouraged me through all the tough years. "I knew you could do it," he responded. Friends, colleagues and children cheered.

Should I bother to call Mom? What possible negative thing could she say about this? Mulling this question over for a couple of days, I determined there was nothing she could say that would be negative about such an exciting prospect for me. Absolutely nothing. So I called her and enthusiastically shared my incredible news.

Her response: "Don't go."

"Don't go? Don't go?" I could not believe she said that.

"You'll just waste all your money going up there."

How deluded could I be, still hoping she might support or encourage me?

Of course I ignored her advice. A year later my book became a resounding success not only in English but also in the Dutch, Swedish and Czech languages. It succeeded in fulfilling my reason for writing it. A survey in the back of my book asked each respondent to state what had been the most helpful thing she learned from reading it. The most repeated response: I discovered my body isn't as bad as I thought it was.

I, the intimidated divorcee, who years earlier could not answer a question in class without tearing up, now appeared regularly on national television as an author and expert, traveling the U.S. and Canada. With the applause of audiences and soaring book sales, the accumulated impact of all of Mom's negative words and actions began to fade. Self-confidence soared. I proved both Mom and my ex-husband were wrong—I could do something right. I turned an idea, a dream, into a product that became successful beyond my wildest hopes. Maybe, I thought, I should give them some credit for my intense drive to succeed. And who knew that creating a silver lining out of all of Mom's criticisms of my appearance would lead to so much fun.

MOM FINALLY TOOK NOTE OF my achievements when she realized how much I traveled around the U. S. and Canada. She came to see us between two of my trips. One afternoon as we sat in the sunroom, enjoying a cup of coffee together and nibbling on some tangy lemon squares, our conversation swung around to my success.

Mom commented, "Diane, you've just been so lucky."

I blinked, then sputtered, "Lucky? Lucky? Let me tell you about luck." Only when I described in detail the six years of research and how I borrowed thirty thousand dollars from the bank to produce and market my workbook, instructor's manuals and videos did her eyes get wide. Mom grew very quiet after my explanation of just how much luck had to do with my success.

"I had no idea," she admitted.

A few months later I appeared as a guest expert on "CBS This Morning." Two of my clients and I demonstrated how the right styles of clothing could camouflage their figure challenges.

Mom, after receiving calls and accolades from her friends about my appearance, called me and said words I never thought I would hear from her.

"Diane, I'm proud of you." That comment stopped me in my tracks.

Mom was proud of me.

Miracles do occur.

After hanging up the phone, I sat still in my rocking chair, gazing out the windows at the ice-covered limbs on the huge maple trees, Mom's words frozen forever in my mind: "Diane, I'm proud of you." Having hoped, wished, wanted and sought her approval for so many years, one would expect me to be thrilled to at last hear her say those words. So thrilled that I might take out a whole page ad in the newspaper proclaiming it, or better yet, a sky-writer to emblazon "Dixie Is Proud of Diane" across the heavens.

Instead, my instant reaction was sadness. Rubbing my forehead with my fingertips, I felt the sadness seeping into my heart. Sad it had taken her the fifty-two years since my birth to give me one compliment. How thrilled I would have been to get any positive comment when younger, especially during those turbulent childhood years. Now I no longer sought her approval. The purgatory of her criticisms had been obliterated by compliments, applause and love from others, especially Rex.

Why did Mom find it so hard to give me a word of praise or encouragement or even a hug all those years? Could it be that she didn't receive them herself as a child?

I recall my uncle remarking, "Growing up as Dixie's brother, trying to meet her high expectations of me was difficult, but I think it has been more difficult for you two girls, growing up as her daughters."

Yes, growing up as Dixie's daughter had been rough. All my life I disappointed Mom—from making a salad, to my looks, to getting a divorce and choosing my career. I always fell short of her expectations. But as her words, "I'm proud of you," echoed in my head again, my mood lightened until a hearty laugh escaped.

Gotcha Mom. You never expected me to become a successful author.

MY NEXT TRIP "HOME" OCCURRED when I went to help Mom through hip replacement surgery.

Early the morning before her surgery, Mom sat on the side of her hospital bed looking woebegone in a wrinkled blue and white floral hospital gown. Grasping my wrist, she gestured toward several items and said, "Now I want you to take my makeup kit to the ICU. Make sure I have lipstick on. And my pretty pink gown and put this pink satin pillow case on the pillow. Sprinkle this scented sachet inside the pillow case." I listened attentively, nodding agreement, but knowing from experience she would not recall a moment of the ICU time, I decided not to bother the staff with her redecorating.

I squeezed her hand, then watched as the orderly wheeled her green draped gurney down the hall and through the wide doors of the surgical suite. A gentle scent of White Shoulders perfume lingered behind.

The whisper of the doors closing didn't give a hint of the mammoth calamity we were about to experience.

18

Questions: Confrontation # 4

MOM'S HIP REPLACEMENT SURGERY WAS a success, but a bad reaction to the anesthesia made her sick for several days. How sick? Sick enough that she didn't care if she had lipstick on. Her intestines shut down and then her electrolytes got fouled up. Unable to keep her lithium down, she became a chemical catastrophe. Asteroids exploded, worlds collided—in her head.

Sitting beside her hospital bed, reading a book, I all but jumped out of my chair as Mom screamed, her voice rising to a shrill pitch "Oh. Oh. OH. KEEP AWAY. SEE THAT MAN? DIANE. OVER THERE BY THE CHAIR. HELP. DON'T LET HIM GET ME. "

Startled, I responded, "Mom, there isn't anyone there," I walked to where she pointed waving my hands through the vacant air.

"HE'S THERE. RIGHT THERE," she sobbed, pointing more to the right, her hand shaking. "He's got on a big, tall black hat. OH STOP HIM. STOP HIM. GET AWAY. GET AWAY."

Nothing could convince her that the scary man was not going to attack her, again and again. It broke my heart to see her cringing, trembling in fright. No amount of consoling calmed her. During the next couple of days she had conversations with other people who were not there, but at least not attacking her.

I had read that during mania some patients experienced hallucinations, but this was the first time Mom had exhibited that symptom. Her medical team kept trying to get her body back on track. They didn't have instant success.

After her hallucinations disappeared, intense agitation set in. Mom became furious at everyone, throwing any reachable item and having

Questions: Confrontation # 4

screaming tantrums. I walked into her room and jumped as a magazine sailed past my legs. When the housekeeper tried to clean around her bed Mom threw a glass of water on her.

"I'm so sorry miss, she doesn't know what she's doing."

"Mom, stop acting like this. You need to apologize," I chided.

Her face contorted in fury. With a cry of exasperation, she threw her last pillow at me.

I moved everything out of her reach until endless tirades were all she could throw.

Mentally and physically exhausted after three days and nights of this, I hired a special night nurse to give me a break.

When I arrived at Mom's room the next morning, feeling refreshed from finally getting a night's sleep, the very tired night nurse handed me Mom's diamond rings. Mom had thrown them at her.

The medical team still could not get her stabilized. I called Gracie to come help. We took shifts watching and trying to calm Mom. That turned out to be impossible. At one point during Gracie's shift, in an awful fit of anger and unable to reach anything else, Mom took out her false teeth and threw them at her.

In her right mind Mom would have been appalled to know the whole hospital staff was buzzing about her bizarre behavior. Thankfully, after about a week, her body started to function better. She started back on lithium. Unfortunately it takes time to be totally effective.

The last day of her hospital stay she became obsessed with the idea that Dad would want her to have a new car, a top-of-the-line car. She called the Lincoln dealership from her hospital bed and arranged to have two cars brought out to her house within an hour of her return home.

"Dad always purchased Buicks," Gracie remarked. "Why a Lincoln and not a Buick?

"Because," Mom declared, wrinkling her nose in disgust, "the Buick salesman had awful halitosis the last time I talked to him."

Hobbling with a walker, her face contorted in pain, Mom tottered back into her latest abode, a house purchased during a manic buying spree the previous year. She plopped down in a dining chair just as two huge Lincoln Town Cars rolled up her driveway: one black, one bronze. Unable to walk out to them, much less drive one, Mom peeked out the window and said, "I'll take the bronze one."

My weary sister and I left her in the skilled hands of a home health team and returned to our respective homes, totally frazzled. The next day Mom fired all the help and called Andrea, who now lived in Ft. Worth, to come help her.

Weeks of rehabilitation passed before Mom's hip healed enough for her to drive her spiffy new car. But once back on her feet, she hit the road—and other things.

I LATER HEARD ABOUT THIS near-death event from Mom's friends, Annie and Jessie. Mom called them and two other friends and offered to drive them in her new Lincoln to a ladies' luncheon given by a mutual friend at her ranch about twenty miles from town. Still a bit manic, talking, not focusing on driving, she drove faster and faster. Careening around a curve, she lost control. The car, racing along the edge of the drainage ditch on the wrong side of the road, threatened to overturn. Her friends screamed. She overcorrected, almost driving the car into the ditch on the other side of the road.

"DIXIE, SLOW DOWN." they yelled. She did, and for a few miles paid attention to her driving, but then, trying to demonstrate the stereo radio, she took her eyes off the road until four frightened voices screamed in unison, "STOP."

Mom looked up, startled. They were racing toward an oncoming car. She swerved with only seconds—and inches—to spare. She apologized and apologized. Her friends, now scared speechless, looked at each other and her.

After the luncheon, when Mom came out of the ranch house, she found Annie firmly planted in the driver's seat. "Dixie, I want to see how this Lincoln drives. I might want one for myself," she said. Nothing Mom could say would budge her friend and they all got home safely.

The word spread. Not one of her friends ever accepted a ride with her again.

THE CYCLE OF STARTING AND stopping lithium didn't end.

"Mom, you need to take your lithium. Why do you keep going off of it? You know what happens," I asked on the phone, my good mood replaced with exasperation.

"I'm okay. I'm fine. I don't need it anymore."

Questions: Confrontation # 4 185

"Yes, you do. You need to start taking it today. Remember what happened last time you stopped it? You got so mad at your health insurance company that you cancelled your policy. Gracie and I had the dickens of a time finding any company that would insure you because of your cancer history. And it's costing you a lot more money than the policy you cancelled."

"Well they made me mad."

Mom had lived without health insurance for six months before we found out. Had her cancer returned, or another major medical problem been diagnosed, her financial security and comfortable lifestyle could have been severely curtailed. Instant anger, followed by impulsive actions, triggered situation after situation that either Gracie or I had to fix.

ONE SUNDAY AFTERNOON MOM CALLED me, interrupting the last three minutes of a March Madness basketball game we were watching. Our team was behind by six points.

"May I call you back in about fifteen minutes after the end of the basketball game we are watching?"

"Well," she insisted, "I need help now."

"Let me change phones." I grimaced at Rex and stomped down the stairs to the sunroom phone.

"What's happened? I asked.

"Well, I don't know who to get to do my taxes," Mom said.

This was her emergency? I sat down with a thud and a huff.

"Why isn't Mike doing them again this year?"

"I got mad and fired him," she said.

Why?"

"He started charging me for phone calls."

"That's what professionals do," I explained, "they charge for their time when you're talking business on the phone." Lordy, how long has she been off lithium this time? She probably made a nuisance of herself, bombarding Mike with a series of irritating calls.

"Well it isn't right. He shouldn't do that," Mom pouted. Your Dad never did. People even called him at night and woke him up."

"I know. He was a wonderful, compassionate doctor. Daddy would want you to take your pills every day so that you don't get so angry at people that you do something that hurts yourself financially. Please, Mom, go get your lithium and take a pill. Right now. Dad would want you to."

Silence on the other end of the line confirmed I had guessed right.

I played the Dad card as often as I thought it would work. Sometimes it did—until Mom decided she was cured—again. I asked myself for the umpteenth time: What will get through to her?

If a medical professional had taken Mom off of lithium, the doctor would have reduced the dosage slowly over weeks, like the time my doctor stopped my thyroid medication. But Mom, on a whim, would just decide one day not to take it anymore and stop abruptly.

I recalled research reporting that manic-depressive illness, left untreated, often worsens over time, with attacks becoming more frequent and more severe. And with repeated gaps in compliance, the medication would become less effective when resumed. Clearly something needed to be done to convince Mom to stay on her pill. But what?

Trying to understand Mom's behavior better, I read more research about bipolar disorder. When manic, she exhibited most of the typical symptoms: heightened mood, grandiose inflated self-esteem, incessant talking, decreased need of sleep, flight of ideas and impulsiveness (like firing her accountant and buying cars). Her erratic driving and spending sprees could also be attributed to mania, as could her explosive anger and whippings when I was a child. But, I wondered, was her screwed up brain chemistry responsible for her constant criticisms even when she was on lithium? Was her disorder the reason she didn't show affection? None of the bipolar information I read included any symptom like "difficulty showing affection."

When manic, Mom believed she had special insight into what was right, and anyone who did not agree with her was absolutely wrong. Unfortunately traces of this characteristic carried over to her more normal periods too. As her years of on-and-off lithium continued, I realized that some of the aberrant behavior she exhibited when in a manic episode reflected just a more virulent version of her basic personality.

AFTER YEARS OF MANIC EPISODES, Gracie and I realized that Mom would continue indefinitely to take us along on the stomach lurching ups and downs of her on-again-off-again manic roller coaster rides. Nothing seemed to stop

Questions: Confrontation # 4 187

her repeating the same scenario, year after year.

Once again I resorted to imagining scenarios with Mom, trying to figure out what actions or words would get through to her. Asking, telling and begging had not worked. What would?

An idea finally popped in my mind. Would it work with Mom?

Prior to my next trip to see her, I rehearsed what I would say. She had to be stable, and on her lithium, for it to work. If she was in the middle of a manic episode, I knew better than to try it. My plan was not to tell, to dictate, or insist or beg that she stay on lithium but to ask her a series of thought provoking questions she would have to answer about why she needed to take that tiny stabilizing pill. We needed her to "own" her problem—and the solution—to accept her illness as ongoing; to accept that her spells would never go away—and to take that pill daily.

Mom waved as I approached the airport luggage carousel. She chatted at a normal pace. Good, I thought, she doesn't seem manic. I claimed my bag and we exited the terminal, looking for the bronze Lincoln, hurrying to get out of the heat.

Does she realize she never touches me, not even for a hello hug?

Observing her carefully all evening and during breakfast the next morning, I determined that not a hint of mania showed.

It's now or never Diane. Do it.

I went to her bathroom and collected her bottle of lithium pills. Even though I had prepared for days for what I was about to do, I entered the living room with a nervous fluttering in my chest. I mentally checked off the series of questions I planned to ask. Holding her lithium pill bottle concealed in my clammy hand, I held onto hope that asking critical questions would get through to her. Gracie and I were more than fed-up with her repetitive noncompliance and the crisis that always followed.

Mom, still in her aqua housecoat, sat at her antique desk, her back to me.

Steeling myself for the task before me, I said, "Mom, I have something serious to discuss with you. Please come over here." She turned and looked at me, tiny eyebrows raised. I patted the seat next to me on the turquoise sofa. Hesitating, she turned and finished writing something, then she rose and moved to sit where I had patted.

188 MOM, MANIA, AND ME

"What's so serious?" she asked, eyebrows still raised.

Taking a deep breath I started my rehearsed script, "Mom, you know that June, your next-door neighbor for years, is diabetic and that she has to have insulin shots every day?"

"Yes." A puzzled look crossed her face.

I continued, "When June's blood sugar spikes, would you, a nurse, advise her to stop her insulin shots?"

"No, of course not."

"Why not?"

"Because she needs them."

"Why does she need them?" Mom didn't answer. A wary look crossed her face.

I asked, "Because the insulin stabilizes her body's reaction to sugar?" I paused, waiting for Mom to nod, then continued, "And what could happen if June chose not to get an insulin shot when she needs one?"

Mom frowned, knowing where this headed, "Well, she could go into a diabetic coma."

"And die?" I asked. She nodded in agreement.

"Mom, you are so lucky." I paused. "So lucky that your imbalance is in your brain and not your pancreas. June has to have insulin shots every day to stabilize her blood sugar. To keep it from getting too high or too low. You also have a chemical imbalance like diabetes, like June's. Only instead of a chemical missing in your pancreas, it's missing in your brain. That's why you are so lucky," I finished with a small smile.

She stared at me, total disbelief registering on her face.

"Yes, you are lucky. To get your chemistry stable all you have to take is one tiny pill, one time a day. Not even one shot. Nor do you have to prick your fingers several times every day and do glucose tests."

I continued with my list of preplanned questions, "Will June's pancreas ever produce the insulin she needs to stabilize the sugar in her blood?"

Mom stared at me, then shook her head.

Then I asked the critical question: "When you quit taking your lithium pills, what has happened within weeks, every time?"

No response. She wouldn't look at me. She looked trapped.

"You have another bout of mania, don't you? Every time Mom. Every time.

Questions: Confrontation # 4

It is tragic that neither June's pancreas nor your brain will ever make the missing chemicals, but at least you won't go into a coma or die from your chemical imbalance. Thank goodness you don't have diabetes."

Mom looked away.

I continued, "Because your brain will never, ever, stabilize itself, you will need to take one lithium pill a day, every day, for the rest of your life—no shots, no pricks, just one small pill."

She still wouldn't look at me.

Sticking to my plan, I played the ultimate guilt card. "I know you don't like to take pills. I also know you have prayed for years for God to help you through your spells. God has answered your prayers. It is in the form of this tiny little pill," I said, holding up her pill bottle. "When you stop taking these pills you are saying 'No' to God. You're rejecting His answer to your prayers."

I let that soak in, the silence remained unbroken between us before I quietly asked, "Mom, please tell me you'll accept God's answer and take your pill every day—every day— for the rest of your life."

She looked at me without speaking. I reached out and placed the bottle of pills in her hand. She looked at it. Looked out the window. Looked down, staring at the pill bottle for a long time, then with a sad smile and small shrug, she nodded.

The next time I saw her friend Jessie, she grinned and related how Mom had told her soon after my visit that she had a problem similar to diabetes, and that she had to take a pill for it. It was the first time Mom had ever admitted to anyone outside the family that she had a problem. Of course, Jessie, and most of the town, had been aware of Mom's manic behavior for over forty years.

Did Mom always take that pill faithfully? No. But she did for many years until elderly when she sometimes forgot it. The change was wonderful. Mom acted normal most of the time. Gracie and I relished the months when only the idiosyncrasies of her personality challenged us.

I just wished I had thought of that diabetes analogy, the religious connection and the list of questions twenty years earlier.

19

Gracie:
Confrontation # 5

EVER SINCE DAD DIED, GRACIE and I had wondered if Mom would ever remarry. Men had gravitated to her all her life, especially during the early days of a manic episode when she playfully flirted. That widower who had come by the house to express his sympathy right after Dad died didn't come through for her, but within a year of Dad's death, another widower, a college president from a nearby town, started courting Mom—until she had cancer. His wife had died of cancer and Mom's bout with it scared him off.

The next widower to try his luck was a fellow from her church. He resided in an apartment next to hers, after one of her many moves. This resulted in knocks on the walls to each other, playing card games together in the evenings and many happy moments for her. Mom didn't seem to care that he had two other girlfriends until he tried to get her to go on a trip with him. She promptly refused. What would people say? So he took another of his lady friends. That ended the knocks on the wall from her side.

MOM'S FREQUENT REQUESTS THAT WE all come home for Christmas resulted in the extended family descending on North Creek one holiday. We gathered at her latest abode, the one-story ranch-style house she had impulsively purchased. She didn't put up a real Christmas tree. Instead, she had a two-foot-tall brass tree with tiny fake, wrapped boxes at the base. At least some Christmas candles and a real pine wreath created the scent of Christmas in the air.

That holiday visit is memorable for two reasons: prairie dogs and worms. The first item involved a video that my college-aged niece and Shannon filmed around the town. Since the military base had closed years

Gracie: Confrontation # 5

191

before, the town had shriveled and all but dried up and blown away. Their scenes of the derelict drive-in movie lot with a few old speakers dangling from rusty posts, and the marquee shot up by the local cowboys, brought back memories of having to leave before the movies were over. The next scene focused on a huge tumbleweed rolling over and over, finally joining piles of the round dried plant that filled parking places at the abandoned burger joint. We teens had circled that building in our cars over and over, hoping to be noticed by certain boys. The film finale panned scores of little mounds of dirt poking up in what had been a prairie dog town on Lookout Mountain.

"Here prairie dog, come on out, little prairie dogs," they cooed over and over as the camera focused on first one empty mound and then another. Not one furry little head popped up. Even the prairie dogs had abandoned the town.

That evening, with eleven of us present, several found places to sit on the floor while we opened our gifts one at a time, sharing the fun of seeing what everyone received: clothes, books, kitchen gadgets and sports equipment. Rex had bought a small fishing pole with a bag of a hundred plastic worms for our grandson, Andrea's four-year-old son. He eagerly ripped open the bag scattering plastic worms everywhere. We started picking them up when suddenly a worm flew through the air. Then another. Soon worms were flying in every direction amid squeals and giggles.

"Stop it. Oh stop this." Mom scolded over our laughter, an ugly frown on her face. About that time a wiggly six-inch plastic worm landed on her lap. She looked at it, gingerly picked it up, got an impish grin on her face and tossed it. By the time the worms stopped flying, we all, including Mom, had laughed ourselves to tears. Our family sharing laughter—the best Christmas gift ever.

THE YEARS SPED BY AND finally, at age eighty-five, Mom made the difficult decision to move to a multi-level care facility in Dallas near Gracie. I went to help her move, one more time.

Sunday, the day after I arrived in North Creek, I awakened to the ringing of nearby church bells. After the morning service, Mom's church had a lovely farewell reception for her. Many old friends came up and told me wonderful things Mom had done for them over the years—giving some furniture to the young assistant pastor's family who didn't have any, visiting another's elderly parent every week for years, and helping a young mother with multiple sclerosis.

Everyone began wishing Dixie the best in her new home when a fellow I had gone to school with pulled me aside and quizzed me, "They say she's taking her car to Dallas. Please tell me this isn't so."

"Why?" I asked, trying to suppress a grin.

He thought a moment and said, "Let me put it like this. God parted the Red Sea for Moses and he parts the traffic for Dixie. When I see her car barreling down the middle of the street at fifty miles an hour, I just pull over to the curb and pray she misses me."

Obviously lithium didn't totally slow her down. Only five months before, she had pulled out onto a highway and hit a car containing a new mother and week-old baby. Luckily the cars were all that were damaged—that time. Gracie and I had been afraid for years that Mom's erratic driving would seriously hurt or even kill someone. Each crash made us worry about the next time—and there would be one. Unable to persuade Mom to stop driving after this latest accident, Gracie and I discussed it and decided it was time to turn Mom into the Texas State Police to be given her first driving test ever. Gracie made the call and tattled on Mom, probably feeling guilty like I did the first time I called Dr. Fisher. But months went by and they never did test her, so it fell to us to dissuade her from driving in Dallas. She hated giving up that car, her mobility, her independence, but finally agreed to do so after she moved to Dallas. She kept getting confused on how to find her way from her apartment to Gracie's house, only twelve blocks and three turns away.

The day of the big move Mom seemed to be having difficulty accepting reality. I couldn't get her to finish packing her suitcase. Knowing if it remained in her bedroom that the movers would put it on the van and she would be without any clothes for several days, I tossed more clothes in, closed it and put it in the trunk of the car.

She also got the strangest look on her face when she decided to fix lunch, opened the cupboards and discovered all the dishes, silverware and pots were missing. We did exchange a grin when the movers picked up the large television console and there, residing under it for several years, were two of those plastic worms.

Gracie: Confrontation # 5

Mom and I watched the moving van pull away and turned back to the empty house. After taking a silent last look around, Mom closed the door and got in the car. We headed over to Annie's to spend the night. Unusually quiet all evening, Mom seemed to be facing the difficulty in saying goodbye to her friends and the town where she had lived since arriving as a bride fifty-six years earlier.

We awakened the following morning to the smell of homemade cinnamon rolls, eggs, bacon and coffee. Annie had prepared a farewell feast.

After hugging our lifelong friends goodbye, with a catch in my throat, I pulled the car away from the curb. As we drove down the familiar streets for possibly the last time, I broached what I planned to do, dubious of how Mom would react.

"Since we don't know when we will ever be back in town, I really want to go by the cemetery to check on Dad's grave." I glanced at Mom and saw the negative shake of her head. I ignored it and kept driving, heading south down the highway. Mom stayed silent.

I parked by the grave site, exited the car and walked toward Dad's grave, ignoring Mom. Finally I heard her car door shut. We stood there in the early morning sunshine looking at the flat metal markers designating the final resting place of her husband and her baby.

I bent down to brush away grass clippings from Dad's marker, running my finger over the still chilly metal letters denoting the beginning and ending of his life. I silently thanked him for his unending support and for the college education that changed my life.

Mom, silent until now, said, "Let's go." She turned and headed to the car, reminding me of the day of Dad's funeral when she had insisted we leave his graveside so abruptly.

I took a last look, rose and followed her, thinking that soon all the people who knew what a caring doctor he had been would also be gone.

We headed toward Dallas. As the miles passed, the terrain changed from land sprouting oil derricks to craggy flat-topped buttes, then to grassy, low rolling hills. Cattle clustered around water troughs under windmills that turned in the brisk wind.

During the drive I asked Mom about selling her house. "Mom, at the church party a man introduced himself as a real estate agent and wanted to know why you didn't respond to his calls after his client made an offer on your house. Did you have two offers?"

"Yes. But I didn't like his buyer as much as the one I sold it to, so I didn't call him back."

I all but moaned. She had two buyers and a possible bidding war over her house and she had accepted the first offer from one of them because she liked him better.

Mom never claimed to have business acumen and had just proven it, but why didn't she call her daughter, the formerly successful real estate agent, and ask my advice? Per usual, she never asked for advice from either Gracie or me. She gave advice, not the reverse.

In Dallas, Mom selected a spacious one-bedroom apartment located in a high-rise building in the independent living section of the multi-level care facility. Being on the first floor proved to have advantages: no wait for an elevator plus a close proximity to the dining hall where she joined other residents for her evening meals. It also had a private patio that contained a large shade tree, and to Mom's delight, a birdhouse with a small feathered resident.

Gracie's daughter came over to help get Mom settled. A veteran mover, she whisked everything into place in a couple of hours. Noting Mom's new beige sofa blending into the all-beige walls she added colorful sofa pillows to relieve the tan tedium. With the kitchen and bath organized, we started hanging pictures and arranging Mom's knickknacks.

Each move I had helped Mom make over the years had called for a reduction in her belongings. Now down to one bedroom and a living-dining area, her choice mementoes remained the trinkets gathered in all her travels to exotic places, plus a large group of many different types of ceramic birds. After my niece grouped the birds together in an attractive display in the mahogany breakfront, Mom, appearing intrigued, said, "I didn't realize I owned so many."

Each day I came by I noticed Mom had rearranged more of her belongings. Her breakfront started to look like the over-crowded display window of a five and dime store, full of every different memento she could possibly cram in there, and her covey of birds were now scattered throughout her apartment. I guess she didn't like having her things arranged by someone else any more than Granny or I did.

Gracie: Confrontation # 5

195

STILL VIVACIOUS AND FLIRTY, MOM had only one thing that slowed her down—a major pain in her right knee. She hobbled everywhere, moving slower and slower. Clearly her knee needed to be repaired. A couple of days after she moved in, Gracie and I were slowly walking with her to the dining room when Mom stopped abruptly. "Look at that. Look at that poor lady." She pointed to a woman. "She can hardly walk." Gracie and I glanced at each other and tried in vain to suppress our grins, because that lady's progress was at least twice Mom's speed.

Why is it we all have so much trouble seeing ourselves clearly?

GRACIE AND I WEREN'T SURPRISED that within a few weeks of Mom's arrival she had a boyfriend. Still attractive, slim and extroverted, she caught the attention of Al, a tall, well-groomed former traveling salesman. Her first date with Al didn't ring any romantic bells. He, still driving at eighty-nine, offered to take her to a pharmacy to get some skids for the legs of the walker she needed after her knee replacement surgery. Soon they were spending their evenings holding hands and watching television, often the Lawrence Welk show. She admitted he had tried to kiss her but she wouldn't let him.

Al fell hard for Dixie. Two months later he asked Mom to marry him, still never having kissed her.

"Are you going to, Mom?" Gracie asked.

"Heavens no. There aren't any sparks there."

Still looking for sparks at age eighty-six. Way to go, Mom.

A FEW MONTHS AFTER MOM'S move to Dallas, Gracie called me to relay what transpired after she noticed Mom getting hyper. All the signs were there: unceasing loud talking, jumping topics, laughing and flirty, not sleeping well. Suspicious, Gracie asked, "Mom, did you stop taking your lithium?

"Yes. I did," she admitted, looking a little guilty, "I'm just taking too many pills. Too many."

"If you didn't want to take so many pills, why didn't you stop taking your thyroid?" Gracie asked.

"Oh, no, I need my thyroid."

"How many years have you been taking thyroid?"

"Oh, forever," Mom said with a shrug.

"And your thyroid gland is still not working normally?"

"No. I need my thyroid pill."

"So, your thyroid pill is a thyroid supplement, not a cure, right? You need to take a thyroid pill every day? Gracie asked.

"Yes."

"And your lithium? What is it? A cure or a supplement?"

Silence. Finally Mom said, "But I don't feel like I need it anymore."

Switching tactics, Gracie asked, "What would happen if you stopped your thyroid?"

Mom didn't reply.

Gracie said, "Your energy would probably feel fine the first few days, like you were cured. But within a couple of weeks you'd start feeling really tired and your hair would begin to fall out." Gracie paused, then added, "What happens within a few weeks every time you stop your lithium?"

Mom stared at her.

"Just like your neighbor June's pancreas never started producing the insulin she needed every day, your thyroid gland won't start producing thyroxin either. Nor will your brain produce the lithium it needs for you to think clearly. Neither your thyroid nor your brain will ever be cured. You have to take both supplements every day. Diane and I need for you to take them both. Will you please do that?"

Gracie reported, "Mom looked sad and her shoulders slumped, but she finally nodded she would."

I have wondered if Mom would have been more compliant if Gracie and I had thought to thank her often when she did take her pill daily. Mom loved and responded to compliments and we should have tried praising her with comments like, "Mom, you're terrific. Thank you for staying on your lithium this month," or, "We are so proud of you, this is the third month you have stayed on your lithium. You are wonderful for doing so." Reinforcing, positive comments possibly could have averted, or delayed, many of her relapses.

THE FOLLOWING YEAR WENT BY peacefully with Mom staying on her lithium, making friends, participating in the many social activities provided in her facility and watching the Welk show with Al.

Then disaster struck.

20

Tragedy, Love, Peace

WORKING ON A WATERCOLOR IN my third floor studio, I was tilting the paper to get the wet red and yellow pigments of a sunset to flow together when the phone started ringing. If I answered, the colors would dry wrong, so I Ignored it. Fifteen minutes later it started ringing again. I swished my brush in the jar of water and on the third ring, picked up the receiver.

"Diane, Diane, it's Gracie," her voice sounded tense, "something has happened to Mom."

"What? What's happened?" I asked, anxiety hitting me in the stomach.

"She's in a coma in the ER. Al found her unconscious on the floor of her apartment. They aren't sure what happened. She's had an upset stomach and has been vomiting and she may have aspirated vomit and passed out."

"What are the doctors saying?"

"It doesn't look good. She's on a ventilator that is breathing for her. I think maybe you should come. They think she may not survive."

Stunned over the news of Mom's condition, adrenaline surged through my body as I went into super-efficient mode, taking care of many business and home tasks before boarding a flight to Dallas a few hours later. My suitcase contained an appropriate dress to wear to Mom's funeral. During the flight, a feeling of helplessness washed over me. There were still so many unresolved emotional issues between us. Why had I waited?

MOM LOOKED SO ILL, HER skin pale. IV's dangling everywhere. A big tube protruded from her mouth. The ventilator made the only sound, swishing as it breathed for her. I tried talking to her, to get any indication that she heard me. Not one movement. No response to a squeeze of her hand. None.

The next day the same stillness, and the day after. And the week after that.

I entered Mom's room in the ICU and once again picked up her hand, stroking it, asking her to squeeze mine. Still no response. I lifted her arms and went through a series of exercises the physical therapist had shown me to keep her limbs and fingers from tightening up. No response.

Pushing a straight backed chair to Mom's bedside, I sat down and looked around. All six beds in Mom's ICU room were now occupied. Two nurses moved silently and quietly among them, monitoring all their patients' vital signs. Hospital sounds echoed down the hall. Beepers beeped. Announcements started and stopped. Green scrub-suited people walked by, pushing patients on gurneys.

I looked at my eighty-six-year-old mother a long time, noticing her graying hair but still fairly smooth skin. Lost in memories for a few moments, I started to quietly talk to her, to tell her goodbye.

The dark haired nurse came over and pulled the green privacy curtain around us.

Holding Mom's hand, I spoke of places she had taken me as a child, how she had helped me when I had my back surgery, and when my children were sick, plus the fun on our cruise. The memories came out in patches—but only good ones. It was the most pleasant conversation we ever had.

AFTER DAYS OF STILL NO improvement in Mom's condition, the doctors explained that even if her body survived, due to the lack of oxygen prior to Al finding her, she would probably be brain damaged and need to go to the full-care unit at her facility. Gracie and I faced the daunting task of clearing out her apartment.

WE ENTERED HER APARTMENT, DRAGGING in a huge stack of flattened packing boxes, rolls of tape and piles of packing paper. Where to start? We divided up the tasks. Gracie started packing the kitchen. My tasks included looking for all documents related to settling Mom's estate and taxes. I opened the dark wooden two-drawer file cabinet I had given her after seeing her bills and critical papers all dumped together in a blue plastic dishpan. Gracie had set up multiple files for her, all carefully labeled. I pulled out the first folder titled "Medicare," opened it and blinked at the first sheet. It stated: Congratulations,

Tragedy, Love, Peace

your Neiman Marcus charge card number is xxxxxx. Good Grief. Evidently, if she stuck a paper in a folder, any folder, it was filed. I would have to go through every page in every folder and both drawers were crammed full.

We boxed, labeled, taped and set aside the items that were designated to be inherited by different family members. They would be shipped out the next day to the recipients.

We started on her closets, jammed with years of outdated clothes, including some polyester pants we were sure could stand up by themselves. We tried to decide what clothes to select for her to be buried in, and selected a lovely pink cashmere outfit, one of her favorites. That went into the small keep-pile with the idea that we should get it cleaned, just in case. Gracie took bags of Mom's clothes over to the office for the administration to disperse to some of the housekeepers and healthcare aides.

Last closet. My back ached as I bent over to look through the stack of flattened boxes and old handbags on the floor. I started to toss some crumpled papers into the trash bag, but a quick glance made me gasp.

"Gracie. Look. Mom has a Health Directive."

We didn't know she had one. Years before when Rex and I had ours drawn up, I suggested Mom do the same. End of conversation. She never mentioned to either Gracie or me that she had one. And what was it doing, loose, in this pile of flattened boxes?

We took it into the living room and sat down next to each other on her beige sofa. Reading Mom's directive, we learned that it was her wish that her life not be sustained on life support equipment. Gracie and I looked at each other. What do we do now? She was on life support—the ventilator.

Taking her directive to the hospital the next morning, we arranged a meeting with the doctors and Chaplain to discuss what to do. The options were limited. Tears flowed as we made a decision no child ever wants to make. They would take Mom off of the ventilator on Friday, two days from now. A tracheotomy would not be done.

We called the rest of the family to come. Mom was going to die Friday.

When Rex arrived the next evening at Gracie's house, he enveloped me in a warm hug for a few moments. As he started to release his arms, I clung on. I craved the security of those broad shoulders, his tender hug, his support and love.

On Friday the staff turned off Mom's ventilator, removed the breathing tube and all IV's. They moved her out of ICU into a private room so we could say our final goodbyes. The family gathered from all parts. We watched Mom for two days, her chest barely moving with each shallow breath, lying so still, so un-Dixie-like. On the third day, her eyelids fluttered. Then opened. She looked at all of us, somewhat puzzled—and tried to smile. Her throat, irritated from the tube, kept her from talking in more than a whisper.

The change in Mom was amazing to behold. An aura of calmness and peace surrounded her. "I love you," she whispered, over and over, to everyone, including Al, including me. It appeared that more than one miracle had happened. Those loving, caring words, so long awaited, were welcomed by all of us. Each time she said them to anyone I felt a lift of my heart, especially when she said them to me. Those three words were like sunshine bursting out after a long, dark storm.

What prompted this loving expression? And the serenity in her face? Had she been with the angels? With God? I didn't recognize this loving, peaceful woman, but hoped she was here to stay.

She stayed about four days. Then the Dixie we knew reappeared.

"What happened to your hair? Put on some lipstick."

Mom's comments about my hair had become a family legend. Each visit, I could count on a derogatory comment about it. On a previous visit several months earlier, when we approached Mom's room for the first time that trip, Shannon, her husband, and Rex took bets on how long it would take Mom to say something negative about my hair.

When we entered her room, Mom looked up. She smiled as we greeted her, looked at me and blurted out, "What have you done to your hair now?" She looked a little puzzled when Shannon called out, "Twenty-six seconds," and we all started laughing. Shannon won the bet that time.

IN THE MONTHS FOLLOWING MOM'S miraculous survival, faced with a physically frail and sometimes mentally confused Mom, I knew my opportunity to broach the sensitive topic of our rocky relationship had passed. I would never know the answer to my questions: Why don't you show me any sign of affection? Why don't you touch me? Do you love me?

Tragedy, Love, Peace

Reflecting on my relationship with Mom led me to consider my other relationships. I too was often remiss in showing affection, even when I felt it strongly. I needed to change my own behavior, to hug more, to start uttering aloud the compliments I too often thought in silence.

AFTER HER SKIRMISH WITH DEATH, Mom went to reside in the full care facility. It took months for her to recover even some of her energy. At first her abilities and memories were garbled, but with time and rehabilitation she regained most of her physical capabilities, a good portion of her memories, and all of her challenging personality. That's when Gracie and I started having trouble evading her questions as to what had happened to her clothes. Mom certainly could recall an amazing number of specific garments that were now missing. Gracie and I were concerned she might one day stop some of the housekeepers and ask them where they got a jacket, or dress that looked just like one she used to have.

Our evasive answers to her frequent inquiries about missing items like her coral colored suite or beige shoes became, "You have such a small closet here we had to put them in storage."

When Mom recovered enough to graduate to the assisted-living unit, she needed to furnish her efficiency apartment with her own belongings. Having shipped furniture and accessories in all directions when we cleared her apartment, we now had to surreptitiously ship some back. She started adding missing decorative items to her inquiries about missing clothes.

"That's in storage too, Mom," we would reply before changing the subject, aware that she would be very upset if she knew we had given away her belongings without her permission.

AFTER HER COMA, I TRIED to get to Dallas twice each year to relieve Gracie of her constant supervision of Mom's needs and demands. Even in an excellent facility, someone needed to see to such things as buying her new underwear, taking her to medical appointments and doing laundry so that her remaining good clothes were not ruined by the facilities' scalding laundry temperature. These tasks fell on Gracie all year around except during my visits when I tried to totally relieve her of all the Mom responsibilities. The result—I typically fell asleep in my plane seat before my flight took off.

While in Dallas I spent hours with Mom. We talked and reminisced, sometimes looking through the large box full of jumbled family photographs she had accumulated over her lifetime. We talked about many things, but I hesitated when it came to unlocking my feelings. I wasn't sure I could get past the hurt, and anger, that still clogged my heart. We still rarely shared a laugh. Or touched. We never had. I always came away feeling sad, sad about the mother I had and the one I now knew I would never have.

As Mom continued to improve she began to engage in the activities in the Assisted Living area. Her spirits picked up. We were able to take her out for lunches and she even took the van to her church on Sundays. Unfortunately, Mom's stay in that unit didn't last even a year. Still somewhat unstable on her feet, she frequently fell. Most of the falls resulted in only bruises until one sent her back to the hospital with a broken pelvis. Once again she returned to the total care unit, this time to stay. Her days were spent watching television and reading her extensive collection of philosophy books or her Bibles. She wore out more than one.

One major benefit resulted from her living in the increased care units: each day a staffer stood by and watched Mom swallow each of her medications, pill after pill, including her lithium. At long last the days of "I'm cured" declarations and manic behavior were over. Unfortunately this steady dose of lithium failed to smooth out all of Mom's personality quirks.

While many memories were gone, Mom clearly recalled that she liked to have her own way. Unfortunately, the beauty shop in the total care unit had only one operator who displeased her. She recalled liking the shop and operators in the independent area and insisted on having her hair done there.

The beauticians there made the mistake of letting her come one time. The next time Mom called for an appointment, they tried to tactfully explain, "We're so sorry but our insurance doesn't allow clients who are not fully ambulatory to come to our salon. You have to go to the salon in your care area."

"What do you mean?"

"We are not allowed to help you out of the shampoo chair and into the other one."

"I can do that myself."

"I'm so sorry Dixie, but it took two of us to help you change chairs when you came. We cannot accommodate you. We could lose our license if you fell."

Tragedy, Love, Peace   203

"I won't fall," said she who was so unstable that she continued to have a regular fall-of-the-week.

A battle of wills developed. Mom started calling daily demanding to get an appointment. They refused over and over. Mom insisted she could navigate between the stations. They rejected her assessment of her abilities—justifiably. Her daily calls became two, then three, then five. The beauticians didn't want to answer their phone in case it was Dixie again. They finally resorted to installing a caller identification system just to screen and not answer calls from her.

Too bad lithium didn't work on stubborn.

Gracie finally had to resort to getting caller ID also. Mom would call her four or five times a day, full of complaints, unhappy about something. Gracie did yeoman's duty ensuring Mom's needs were met.

If the Baptist church had saints, I'd nominate Gracie.

DURING THE FOLLOWING YEARS, AS Mom became weaker, taking her anywhere became more than I could manage by myself. That eliminated her favorite trips to nearby restaurants that offered her a respite from the repetitive food in her facility. Taking her to a fast-food drive-in became my only recourse. Even though we would stay in the car and not be seen by anyone, Mom still took pride in her appearance. It would take her almost an hour to get ready to go as she chose one outfit, then rejected it for another. After applying full makeup, a dab of White Shoulders and brushing her hair (only in the front), the staff would wheel her to the front door and assist me in getting her into the car. Off we would go to a nearby drive-in for a juicy hamburger plus two of her favorite items—onion rings and ice cream. Pure glee lit up her face each time she bit into her first crisp onion ring. That glee, plus the grin that followed the first spoonful of her chocolate ice cream, made all the effort worth it.

As Mom's ability to get around became more challenging, Gracie and I discussed purchasing her a motorized wheel chair. But standing there in the wide, carpeted hallway, looking at the turtle pace of her elderly colleagues tottering down the hall with their walkers and envisioning Mom motoring at full speed helter-skelter, nixed that idea.

THE NEXT YEARS WERE HEART breakers. Mom shrunk in height to a tiny figure with a rounded back. Mild shaking from Parkinson's became evident.

Her vision and hearing declined. Conversations were full of long silences. Gone was the chatter, the vivaciousness, the extrovert, the take-over and take-charge Mom. Her chief frustrations, her main complaints contained comments that she felt useless, no good, unable to help anybody.

Her frustration began to help me comprehend that it was by doing things for others that my mother showed she cared.

Gracie helped me understand this method of communicating love more fully when she shared some insights into what happened when she and her husband exchanged greeting cards, especially valentines. Each was disappointed in the cards selected by the other. It seemed Gracie wanted to receive sweet poetic cards from her husband. Instead he gave her silly joke cards. He preferred joke cards and got lovey-dovey ones from her. She gave him the type of card she wanted to receive herself, not considering what he preferred, and vice-versa.

The communication specialist in the pre-marital course Gracie and her husband developed for their church explored this Catch 22 with engaged couples. After taking a communication test based on Dr. Gary Chapman's book, *The 5 Love Languages,* the couples often discover that how they express love isn't the same way their partner does. For example, one woman thought the best way to feel loved by her partner was for him to tell her he loved her; her partner had selected doing things for her as the best way to show he loved her. Others stated that loving gestures like hugs, hand holding or tender touches showed love better than just saying loving words. This discussion of how one communicates love made it obvious that the way one person chooses to express loving feelings to another may not meet the emotional needs of the recipient.

I mulled this information over and realized that Mom chose actions to show that she cared. I began to see her love in the things she had done for me. Taking me to events, buying all those clothes, the cruise and helping pay for college for my children were all loving gestures to me. Just not the loving touches I craved from her.

As a child, I sensed that a quick hug or an occasional word of praise, even an encouraging smile, would have made a tremendous difference in my feeling that Mom did love me, even when I didn't do things the way she expected. Receiving things like clothes and trips, did not meet my emotional needs.

All my life Mom's words had reprimanded me, criticized me, hurt me. Her harsh whippings when I was a child devastated me. I needed loving gestures to replace those painful memories—hugs and touches and tenderness that expressed any feeling of her love for me. While Dad had not been overtly affectionate, his occasional hugs without all the negative, harsh criticisms were all I had needed to feel loved by him.

Some members of my writing critique group revealed their personal experiences about how their parents had expressed love. One member shared that while she had received loving hugs from her mother, the positive impact of them was erased by harsh verbal abuse that wiped out the feeling she was loved. A male in the group recalled harsh whippings with a switch, but his Dad's many caring gestures and words at other times made him feel loved.

We must all have our own unique love receptors that need to be met to feel loved. But how will our loved ones know what gestures we need unless we tell them—or show them? How will we know what their emotional needs are unless we observe how they show love, or ask them, "What makes you feel loved? Words? Hugs? Doing things for you? Tell me the best way to show you that I love you."

I FINALLY BEGAN TO LET go of my long-held resentments against Mom in my head and in my heart. At this stage of her life, confronting her would serve no purpose. She probably had no memories of my childhood whippings or her endless criticisms, and no idea how deeply her actions had wounded me. Studies show that mammals (including people) who are not cuddled and nurtured as babies and youngsters do not turn into nurturing parents. I suspect that may be a reason I turned out to be a mother who, while craving loving gestures myself, didn't give an abundance of them to my own children. I realize that my intense feelings for my children, while felt internally, have not been expressed overtly often enough.

When I look back and wonder why Mom found it so hard to show any physical affection to me, I now suspect she didn't get many hugs, compliments, or encouragements when a child either.

My attitude toward Mom changed as I began to look at her more objectively. I realized that my first impression, my earliest memories of her, were of Scary Mom. The memories of the screaming, the harsh whippings, created the dark lens through which I viewed her all my life. They had distorted and magnified her faults to the point of stifling any acknowledgment that she had expressed love and caring through her many positive actions toward me and my family. My lifetime view of her had been obscured and warped by the abusive events that happened before I turned eight years old.

I now acknowledged that Mom had dealt with a chemical imbalance in her brain all her life that created havoc in her mind, in her actions, in her life—and ours—yet she had managed to be a productive person, making a positive difference in many lives. She had risen from poverty, educated herself and others, been an asset in her church and community—and in her own way, a loving parent.

Mom didn't have a choice in becoming bipolar-manic. No one knows what causes this chemical challenge. Acknowledging this helped loosen the resentments I had sustained over all these years.

As her life began to fade away, so did my hurt and anger.

AFTER THINKING ABOUT OUR EMOTIONAL challenges, I knew Mom wouldn't, couldn't, change her ways, but I could change mine. She didn't give hugs, but I could. I wanted to share my preferred sign of affection—a tender, caring hug—with her. Thus I began initiating a hug with Mom during the last moments of my visits to Dallas. Just before I left I would reach out to help her stand up from her beige recliner. Each time she looked puzzled and asked, "Why, what are we going to do?"

"I want to hug you, Mom," I would say as I encircled my arms around her short, stooped body and gently held her for a few moments before leaving to return to my home. I repeated this last-minute ritual every visit for several years.

During Mom's ninety-second year, as dusk fell at the end of the first day of my week-long visit, I stood up, preparing to go to Gracie's where I was to stay. Mom started struggling to stand up.

"What do you want to do Mom?" I asked.

"I want to hug you."

I blinked. Mom wanted to hug me.

I bent over and placed my hands under each of her arms. Slowly lifting her to her feet, I struggled to support her full body weight. She tottered, then

Tragedy, Love, Peace 207

steadied as she reached out her arms to embrace me. Our arms encircled each other. Her head came to rest on my shoulder.

How tiny and frail she had become.

I felt her arms slowly tighten around my ribs. Tighter. Tighter. I felt my heart beating once again against her cheek, as it had so many years ago. I felt her love totally envelop me. We clung to each other for a long time in this gesture of love and caring.

I wanted that hug to last forever. The memory of it has.

ON THE LAST DAY OF my visit, I didn't have a chance to give Mom my usual goodbye hug. My last sight of her, before leaving to catch my flight, included the visiting dentist bending over her in bed, about to extract a broken tooth.

A week after my return home, just as I pulled back the covers to crawl into bed one night, the phone rang. It was Gracie. After an evening out, she and her husband had stopped by to check on Mom who appeared to be failing in the past few days. Already in bed, Mom stirred, recognized her and said, "Thank you for coming."

As Gracie sat by the bedside holding Mom's hand, she watched her drift off to sleep. Shortly, Gracie realized that Mom's finger tips had begun to turn cold. She kept holding her hand, stroking it and patting her arm until with a soft sigh Mom released her last breath.

Mom died, looking peaceful and relaxed, a state of being denied to her, and us, so much of her life.

Epilogue

WRITING THIS BOOK HAS BEEN a rocky journey. I had to stop writing at times, especially when my critique group asked a question that sent my mind reeling: "Where was your Dad when your mother was whipping you? Why didn't he stop her?" After searching my memory and conferring with Gracie, I realized that Mom never whipped me when Dad was around. Nor did she lose her temper anywhere but in the privacy of our home.

My Dad never knew. I never told him. He never asked.

Young children have no choice but to tolerate mistreatment by adults. The place a child feels the most fear of an abusive parent is the exact place the parent feels the safest to abuse the child—in the privacy of their home.

When I realized this, I had to deal with renewed anger toward Mom. Yes, she had a mental illness that may have been the cause of her flashes of fury, but evidently she could, and did, control when and where she lost control.

While I hope that my story is not typical of what happens to every child of a parent with mental illness, physical and emotional abuse does occur. Another example: one evening Rex and I went to a neighbor's home for dinner. Dawn, our hostess, appeared agitated. She finally blurted out the reason, disgust in her voice, "My parents arrive later tonight. My mother is bipolar and she won't stay on her meds."

Our ensuing conversations revealed we had similar experiences—and responses.

"My mother would get instantly mad," she said, "one minute she was fine, the next furious. The worst thing she ever did to me when I was little was grab me by my long hair and throw me across the room. I eloped at 19 to get away from her."

Why I Wrote *Mom, Mania, and Me*

- to impress upon family members and counselors that young children with an unstable parent need help to cope with what they cannot understand, control, change or escape;
- to explain that a person who has an imbalance of a chemical in their brain didn't have a choice. It isn't their fault and no amount of their will power, nor your love, will cure it;
- to encourage anyone who even suspects that they, or a loved one, may have mood instability to seek medical help from a physician who specializes in mood disorders; and
- to let others know that having a negative relationship in your life does not mean you have to have an unhappy life.

What I Learned as a Child of a Bipolar Parent

- One can survive and thrive. In fact, the impact of the parent's negative behavior can become the catalyst for your drive to succeed.
- Many bipolar patients reject either their diagnosis or their medication, or both. The comparison of Mom's bipolar problem to diabetes and hypothyroidism helped her accept her illness and stay on her medication.
- Like Mom, a bipolar patient will probably not communicate to a doctor all the critical information necessary for a correct diagnosis. The family needs to confer with the physician also. They need to reveal all mood and physical symptoms they have observed.
- Select a doctor the family can call when help is needed. This is vital in helping the patient, and the family, through difficult times.

Note: Permission for anyone other than the patient to contact the doctor about the patient's care must be arranged under the HIPAA privacy policy. You can independently consult with a psychiatrist, psychologist, mental health counselor or social worker to ask for help for your own needs, and most of all—the needs of the children.

Appendix

Facts & Data
About Mental Illness

THE FOLLOWING INFORMATION IS COMPILED from literature from the following organizations unless otherwise noted:

Depression and Bipolar Support Alliance (DBSA)

The Agency for Health Care Policy and Research (AHCPR) Depression Guideline Panel

The National Institute of Mental Health (NIMH)

National Alliance on Mental Illness (NAMI)

Population Affected by a Variety of Mental Disorders
Approximately 61.5 million adult Americans experience some form of mental illness in a given year. Approximately 18.1 percent of American adults–about 42 million people–live with anxiety disorders, such as panic disorder, obsessive-compulsive disorder (OCD), post-traumatic stress disorder (PTSD), generalized anxiety disorder and phobias.

Youth
One-half of all chronic mental illness begins by the age of 14; three-quarters by age 24. Approximately 20 percent of youth ages 13 to 18 experience severe mental disorders in a given year. For ages 8 to 15, the estimate is 13 percent.

Major Depression
Approximately 6.7 percent of American adults–about 14.8 million people–live with chronic depression.

Schizophrenia
Approximately 1.1 percent of American adults– about 2.4 million people–live with schizophrenia.

Bipolar

Approximately 2.6 percent of American adults (5.7 million people) have bipolar disorder.

Bipolar Disorder Information

Bipolar Disorder

(Affective Mood Disorder; Manic-Depression; Mental Illness)
Bipolar disorder is a treatable physical illness marked by extreme changes in mood, thought, energy and behavior. It is not a character flaw or a sign of personal weakness.

People with bipolar disorder experience unusually intense emotional states that occur in distinct time periods called "mood episodes."

Each mood episode represents a drastic change from a person's usual mood and behavior. The extreme changes in energy, activity, sleep and behavior are described as either manic or depressive episodes. Episodes can last for hours, days, weeks or months.

Symptoms of Mania - The "Highs" of Bipolar Disorder

- Heightened mood, exaggerated optimism and self-confidence
- Excessive irritability, aggressive behavior
- Decreased need for sleep without experiencing fatigue
- Grandiose thoughts, inflated sense of self-importance
- Racing speed, racing thoughts, flight of ideas
- Impulsiveness, poor judgment, easily distracted
- Reckless behavior (author's note: sexual, financial, drugs, alcohol...)
- In the most severe cases, delusions and hallucinations.

Symptoms of Depression - The "Lows" of Bipolar Disorder

- Prolonged sadness or unexplained crying spells
- Significant changes in appetite and sleep patterns
- Irritability, anger, worry, agitation, anxiety
- Pessimism, indifference

- Loss of energy, persistent lethargy
- Feelings of guilt, worthlessness
- Inability to concentrate, indecisiveness
- Inability to take pleasure in former interests, social withdrawal
- Unexplained aches and pains
- Recurring thoughts of death or suicide

Source: The Depression and Bipolar Support Alliance (DBSA)

Testing for Bipolar Disorder

At this time there is no single test to confirm a diagnosis. As most patients do not exhibit all of the symptoms in the previous lists, making a precise diagnosis of bipolar disorder is challenging.

Causes of Bipolar Disorder

There is no single, proven cause or gene that results in bipolar disorder. Research strongly suggests that it is often an inherited biochemical problem related to the lack of stability in the transmission of nerve impulses in the brain.

Genetic Links

Researchers have identified a number of genes that may be linked to this disorder. If one parent has bipolar disorder and the other parent does not, there is a 1 in 7 chance that their child will develop it. The chance may be greater if the families have a number of relatives with bipolar disorder or depression.

Age

Symptoms of bipolar disorder often appear during the late teens and early twenties. Fifty-nine percent of patients with manic depression reported symptoms of their illness during or before adolescence; however, half did not receive assistance for their illness for five years or more.

Children

The symptoms of bipolar disorder resemble symptoms of Attention Deficit Hyperactivity Disorder (ADHD). Bipolar disorder is often misdiagnosed as ADHD. Fifteen percent of children with ADHD may have bipolar disorder. New research shows that a Functional Magnetic Resonance Image (fMRI) can determine the difference between ADHD and Bipolar Disorder in children.

Male vs Female

Women are twice as likely as men to experience depression, while manic depression affects the sexes equally. Men are more likely to start with a manic episode; women with a depressive episode.

Frequency of Episodes

The average person with bipolar disorder has four episodes during the first 10 years of the illness.

Length of Episodes

Episodes can last days or months, or fluctuate over a year. On average, without treatment, manic or hypomanic episodes last a few months, while depressions often last well over 6 months.

Thyroid Connection

While thyroid disease and manic-depressive illness are two entirely separate disorders, and one certainly does not cause the other, there is possibly a connection in some people.

Suicide

People with severe, untreated depression have a suicide rate as high as 15 percent. The risk is highest in the initial years of the illness. Before the late 1970's when the drug lithium first became widely available in the United States, one person in five with manic-depression committed suicide.

Alcohol and Drugs

Forty-one percent of people with bipolar disorder abuse alcohol or drugs when their illness is not being successfully managed, compared to 13 percent when the illness is being managed. At least one-third of all people with bipolar disorder also have comorbid substance abuse.

Source: Dr. Michael Thase, University of Pittsburgh School of Medicine

Family Support

Supportive relationships with family members (including spouses) are key to the daily management of manic depression, according to 90 percent of people surveyed.

Cost to Society

Bipolar disorder devastates family and work relationships and costs society more than $16 billion a year through medical bills, missed work and lower productivity.

Bipolar Disorder vs Schizophrenia

A study of 252 subjects using functional brain imaging (fMRI) compared the interactions between 5 specific brain network systems in three groups of people: persons without psychiatric illness, persons with clear-cut bipolar disorder and persons with clear-cut schizophrenia.

The results indicate there are certain brain network interactions that are uniquely out of balance in bipolar disorder. Other network interactions are uniquely out of balance in schizophrenia. However, there are some interactions that are similarly out of balance in both schizophrenia and bipolar disorder. Source: S. A. Meda and colleagues, *Biological Psychiatry*, 2012.

Bipolar Disorder
Information and Resources

B IPOLAR DISORDERS AFFECT NOT JUST the person afflicted with it, but all who love them, know them, work with them—an estimated 30 million people daily. Families bear the hardest burden. The dread of another manic or depressive episode is a constant concern. We often feel helpless to do anything to either avert an episode or help them through it.

The patient affected by bipolar disorder needs to see a psychiatrist or physician who specializes in mood disorders and is licensed to prescribe medications. The family can benefit from seeing a psychologist, counselor or social worker who specializes in family counseling. Contact the following national health organizations for information on the services near you.

The Depression and Bipolar Support Alliance (DBSA)

The DBSA holds conventions and conferences, operates a bookstore, publishes a newsletter and participates in national campaigns. Medical definitions, methods of treatment, medication data, warning signs and support groups are a major function of local DBSA chapters. This organization, headquartered in Chicago IL, has an excellent web site that includes helpful suggestions for families and friends.

Phone: 800-826-3632

Website: www.dbsalliance.org > Help Others > Friends & Family Center

The National Alliance of Mental Illness (NAMI)

NAMI offers online and Facebook educational courses about mental illness. They are also active with blogs, twitter, advocacy and support groups in every state in the US plus parts of Canada, Mexico and Puerto Rico.

Phone: 800-950-6264 or 703-524-7600

Website: www.nami.org

National Mental Health America (NMHA)

NMHA is a non-profit national mental health association. It assists people with mental illness and their families to find treatment, support groups, medication information and help with issues such as financial concerns for treatment.

Phone: 1-800-969-6642
Website: www.nmha.org

The National Network of Adult and Adolescent Children of Mentally Ill Parents (NNAAMI)

NNAAMI, based in Australia, supports children, young people, and adults around the globe who are coping with mentally ill parents. The website posts articles, advice and forums that are managed by and for the affected group.

Website: www.nnaami.org

Canadian Mental Health Association (CMHA)

CMHA is a nationwide, voluntary organization with provincial branches across Canada. They provide a wide range of innovative services for people who are experiencing mental illness and their families. These services are tailored to the needs and resources of the communities where they are based. One of the core goals is to help people with mental illness develop the personal tools to lead meaningful and productive lives.

Phone: 613-745-7750
Website: www.cmha.ca

The Mood Disorders Society of Canada (MDSC)

The MDSC's overall objective is to provide people with mood disorders with a strong, cohesive voice at the national level and to improve access to treatment, inform research, and shape program development and government policies. MDSC has taken a lead proactive role in public policy and program development with the goal of improving the quality of life for people affected by mood disorders.

Phone: 519-824-5565
E-mail: info@mooddisorderscanada.ca
Website: www.mooddisorderscanada.ca

Mental Health America (MHA)

MHA is the nation's leading community-based nonprofit dedicated to addressing the needs of those living with mental illness. Affiliates provide public education, information and referral, support groups, rehabilitation services as well as socialization and housing services to those confronting mental health problems They bring together mental health consumers, parents, advocates and service providers for integrated care and treatment with recovery as the goal.

Phone: 800-969-6642

Website: www.mentalhealthamerica.net

For the Latest Scientific Research on Bipolar Disorder

The National Institute of Mental Health (NIMH)

NIMH is part of the National Institutes of Health (NIMH), a component of the U.S. Department of Health and Human Services, the world's leading biomedical research organization. The mission of NIMH is to transform the understanding and treatment of mental illnesses through basic and clinical research, paving the way for prevention, recovery and cure. It is the largest scientific organization in the world dedicated to mental health research.

Website: www.nimh.nih.gov

A Conversation with
Author Diane Dweller

Q. What tips can you share about the emotional impact of writing a memoir about painful events?

A. Recalling the trauma of my childhood created deep anguish, pain and anger that overwhelmed me at times. At one point I stopped writing for over two years. It was the compelling drive to help other families challenged by bipolar disorder that propelled me to try again. If writing about hard times creates a crisis, stop. Take a break. Regroup. Then try again.

Q. Did you find writing the book cathartic for you?

A. Absolutely. I am now at peace with my memories of Mom. My angst is gone.

Q. What lessons have you learned from your experience?

A. I learned that you cannot change anyone else. You can change only yourself, your reactions to others and what may happen in the future. You cannot change the past. It is very liberating to let go of it.

Q. How did you select which events to include in your book?

A. I noted on separate file cards each event I thought would be pertinent to the themes of my story. I reorganized those cards until the events flowed in the sequence I wanted. After the first draft was complete, multiple revisions, including multiple deletions, followed.

Q. Studies of memories show that they may become distorted. How did you verify your memories?

A. While siblings rarely recall family events exactly the same way, Gracie did confirm that Mom whipped me, but not as often as I recalled. Gracie, however, was in school during the months following Mom's worst spell after losing the baby. I was home alone with Scary Mom.

We recall highly negative events more vividly than calm or pleasant events. Even if my earliest memories of being whipped frequently as a five year old child were magnified in my mind, my goal to get away from Mom continued until I married at age seventeen. While Mom's behavior did improved after Dad took her for a mental evaluation when I was six, the list I found stating what I would not do as a mother was written after I learned cursive about age eight. I kept and moved this list to our new house when I was ten, thus, some of Mom's devastating behavior must have continued.

Q. Do you have a fear of becoming bipolar like your mother?

A. While bipolar disorder has a genic link that affects one in seven offspring, my sister and I are fortunate that we did not inherit this illness. Symptoms often become obvious during the maturing of the pathways in the brain between the late teen years and early adulthood. We are well past that. Note: Bipolar Disorder occurs only when several genes are defective, not just one.

Q. Looking back, how do you think your experiences molded you, both good and bad?

A. Years of negativity from Mom, and then my first husband came close to destroying my last ounce of self-esteem. As I gained confidence in college, their past put-downs fueled a drive in me to succeed in both my professional and personal life. When negative situations arise now, my first instinct is still to withdraw and stay silent, but when I decide to take a stand—I'm tough.

Q. Are there better diagnostic tools for bipolar disorders now?

A. Yes. Functional Magnetic Resonance Imaging (fMRI) shows brain functions differ in bipolar patients. They also show that the brain shrinks in size when bipolar disorder is not treated or when patients stop taking lithium. Resuming lithium reverses the atrophy and the fMRI shows that the brain expands again. While diagnosing bipolar disorder may now become easier, the challenge of keeping a patient on medication remains.

Q. Did you receive any unexpected insights while writing your memoir?

A. Plenty. One not mentioned in the book is that after writing about hiding in rooms that had two doorways that allowed me to escape from Scary Mom, I walked through the house I designed decades later. I was stunned to realize that every room, except one powder room, had two doorways.

Book Club
Discussion Questions

1. Diane's early feelings toward her mother were not positive. How did they change? What caused the changes?

2. There is a stigma to mental illness. Has this book changed your attitude toward those afflicted with a mental illness?

3. After the cake cutting incident with Shannon, Diane confronted her mother about her criticisms. What do you think would have been the result if she had used the angry tactics she thought about all night? How do you think Dixie would have responded?

4. The author tried to get rid of negative memories in an unusual way. Discuss what she did. How effective was it? What methods have you tried?

5. Diane's behavior as a mother mirrored Dixie's until she found her childhood list. What positive or negative behaviors do you, or a sibling, exhibit that is like one of your parents?

6. Hugs, rather than words, make Diane feel loved. What actions or words make you feel loved?

For More Discussion Questions and to contact Diane,
go to dianedweller.com.

Acknowledgments

N O WRITER WRITES ALONE EVEN though hours alone are needed to produce a manuscript. It is the people who support our endeavor that make our writing time possible and productive. Many special people have helped me along this journey.

I encourage writers to join a writing critique group. The members of the first group I joined were all published authors. A later group included some beginning authors. All contributed to an improved manuscript. I appreciate each comment, each suggestion, each word of encouragement, and yes, each suggestion to change, add or delete words.

My family knows what I owe to each of you for your contributions and support. I acknowledge all of you in my heart, especially Gracie who read the manuscript more than once.

Rex, you stood by me through all my tears and frustrations and cheered me on through the heartbreaking challenge of recalling stressful events. Thank you for being my sweetheart, my supporter, my rock.

Thank you, readers, for your support. I hope you will share the information you found helpful in *Mom, Mania, and Me* with others in challenging relationships.

CPSIA information can be obtained
at www.ICGtesting.com
Printed in the USA
LVHW050140140120
643551LV00011B/666/P